A Theology of Beasts

Also By J. Aaron Gruben

Veterinary Books

Fuzzy Logic: How to Think Like a Veterinarian

Fuzzy Logic 2: How to Keep Thinking Like a Veterinarian

A Theology of Beasts: Christians and Veterinary Medicine

Animal Anatomy Coloring and Activity Books (Canine & Feline)

Chivalry School Studies

Chivalry: An Ancient Code for Our Time (high school to adults)

Chivalry: A Study for Little Knights (elementary)

Bible Study

King: A Christian's Call to Imitate Christ's Kingship

The Tangled Eons Series

Crescent Tides

Fatal Fogs

The Stalwart Supinator: Servant of the Streets!

The Medieval Muddles

Juvament!: A Mythical Mess

The Mubblefubbles: A Toothy Tangle

Children's Books

Elye of Saint Gilles: A Chanson de Geste Retold (Middle grades)

Heaps of Hobs: A Fun-Filled Fable in Old English Verse (Picture Book)

A Theology of Beasts: Christians and Veterinary Medicine

J. Aaron Gruben, DVM

Printed in the United States of America

First Edition, 2021

ISBN 978-1-7339105-7-6

Post Tenebras Lux Books

www.nmgrubens.com
www.posttenebrasluxbooks.com

The author would like to thank

Joy, his incredible wife, who has put up with years of disgusting, case-related dinner conversation and depressing, case-related work stress: all in the service of veterinary medicine.

Ray and Kathy, his wonderful parents, who (as soon as they realized they couldn't talk him out of it) encouraged him on the path to a veterinary career.

Benjamin Keil, brilliant philosopher extraordinaire, whose help in the philosophy section of this book was invaluable.

Table of Contents

Introduction

Hordes of people want to be veterinarians, enough that veterinary schools have difficulty accommodating them. But few consider the full extent of the cost involved.

Counting Up the Costs

I'm not talking about the mere money it takes, though that is a much bigger roadblock than most potential veterinary students understand. The expense of a veterinary education today is so high that the investment for most has to be a lifelong one. Few veterinary graduates can afford the luxury of changing careers.

The academic cost is also high. I found veterinary school to be deceptively difficult. The semester would invariably start with me saying, "Wow! This is simple stuff" and then would end with me pulling out my hair in a frenzy, trying to comprehend the bewildering details of the coagulation cascade, and moaning over the sheer mountains of things I had to memorize.

The emotional cost is likewise high, both during vet school and even more so out of school. When I went to school, the suicide rate among vet students had become alarming enough to justify a permanent counselor on staff. This has only become worse. Recently NBC News reported, "Research has consistently shown for more than 30 years that veterinarians are at significantly higher risk of suicide than is the general population, owing to a combination of factors that include occupational stress, depression and burnout."[i] The article cites a study reporting that 11,620 veterinarians killed themselves from 1979 to 2015.

Part of the reason for this book, however, is to address the even higher spiritual cost of veterinary medicine—a subject certainly not spoken about in veterinary school.

This book is written mainly to Christian veterinarians and potential Christian veterinarians. Some of the topics I hope to cover are the spiritual and deeply-rooted philosophical struggles we face in this field. Modern, materialistic thinking about animal-kind and their relationship to humankind is antagonistic to the Christian viewpoint. And (though it may come as a surprise to some) non-Christian ways of thinking about animals raise an array of practical problems for the practitioner striving to navigate a confusing philosophic landscape.

The Most Important Question

In light of all the costs, is work in the field of animal medicine worth the effort, expense, and risk?

That's a complex question, with a complex answer that varies based on an individual's life circumstances. But for a Christian, the most important part of weighing a costly decision like this is asking whether or not this is a profession he or she can glorify God in. Is this a career that pleases God, and that a Christian can work in honorably?

Even from an early age, we are trained to think of our job on one hand and our Christian life on the other, as if serving God were an after-thought or a hobby we do on our days off from real life at the job. We don't ask, "What do you want to do when you grow up?" as often as, "What do you want to *be* when you grow up?" But Scripture teaches something different. It tells us every part of our lives is supposed to be a means to glorify God. *"So, whether you eat or drink, or whatever you do, do all to the glory of God"* (1 Corinthians 10:31). We should be *all* about the kingdom of Christ. Shouldn't that also include the career we spend so many hours at?

"Animal welfare and health is something the Bible speaks to, and so it becomes a theological question which should shape Christian orthopraxy (how we live in light of doctrine)."

Everyone: Read This Book

You may be a parent of a potential vet student or a friend of a veterinarian. I'd urge you to read this book to become more informed in your discussions with them. Whether the profession of veterinary medicine is God-honoring is a question seldom asked, though is vitally important for many people.

Even if you have no interest in becoming a veterinarian, you probably have a pet or two. That makes this an important topic. You need to know that *"Whoever is righteous has regard for the life of his beast"* (Proverbs 12:10a), and you need to know why. God cares about animal disease and suffering and wants his people to care too. This is the most important reason we should consider the question as Christians.

Animal welfare and health is something the Bible speaks to, and so it becomes a theological question that should shape Christian orthopraxy (how we live in light of doctrine). That's a surprisingly difficult thing for some Christians to understand, and so the question "Is veterinary medicine a noble profession?" is important to every Christian pet owner, agriculture worker, animal caretaker, or human who comes into contact with an animal during their lifetime.

And it's a question that many Christians over the centuries have already answered with their lives' work. The history of veterinary medicine as a professional career, especially at its inception, is an account made up largely of the stories of Christian men and women convinced that the domain of animal health is a calling God cares about. We'll spend the first part of this book learning some of their fascinating stories.

So dive in with me! Come ponder the field of veterinary medicine from the light of the Christian faith. Come learn how Christians have influenced veterinary medicine since its foundation and discover why they thought it an honorable vocation of a follower of Christ.

– I –

Christians and the Development of Veterinary Medicine

If the practice of Veterinary medicine is important for Christians, one would expect to find many Christians involved in the work of animal medicine throughout history. This should be especially true of the formative years of veterinary medicine when practitioners were thinking carefully through the ideals behind animal health, and specifically working to raise veterinary medicine to the status of a respected profession. If the church has reason to care about animal medicine, its involvement should be clear in those developing years in particular. And this is exactly the testimony of history!

"Christians who were vocal about their faith played vital roles in veterinary medicine's development."

People of diverse religious backgrounds ultimately built modern veterinary medicine but, as in human medicine, Christians who were vocal about their faith played vital roles in its development. Even beyond the individuals involved, Christian ideals transmitted through general Christian cultures played a role in developing a concern for animals and an interest in medical theory.

In this section, we'll dig into a fascinating chapter of history rarely studied, and meet some of the many followers of Jesus involved in the excellent work of raising interest in animal wellbeing from a mere hobby to a scientific discipline. They did this because they deemed it important work, because they were convinced of an important need, and because they saw a way to serve Christ that others had overlooked.

What follows outlines the rise of veterinary medicine from a denigrated hobby practiced by a scorned few, to a respectable profession. Remember, as you read the "dry" facts of history, that they are the highlights of the real-life stories of amazing men and women, who lived normal lives and went beyond them to do great things. Always engage your imagination when you read history! The stories are about people who, in the context of a world where even human medicine was primitive and often looked down on, were brave enough to show their care for the animals that surrounded them.

Ancient Medicine

The origin of the word veterinarian is hazy with the mists of the past but may have come from *veterinarium*, a Latin term used in ancient Rome for a building keeping pack animals. Alternately it might have derived from *souvetaurinarii*, the Roman word for those who tended the animals that were sacrificed to tell the future (a practice called haruspicy).[ii]

The ancient Romans practiced veterinary medicine, but it seems to have been more empiric (based on observation and guesses), rather than based on scientific studies and literature. It borrowed medical theory from the Greeks, who were more advanced in philosophy and writing about medicine. This contrast between the empiric, practical nature of Roman veterinary medicine and the more scholarly Greek practice of veterinary medicine is a dichotomy we'll see throughout the field's history. It was a dichotomy effectively bridged in the Byzantine veterinarians in the medieval period.

Byzantine Veterinarians

Byzantium was a continuation of the eastern half of the Roman Empire after Rome succumbed to Germanic tribes in the 5th century. It remained a mighty empire for a thousand years until 1453, the year the Ottoman Turks took Constantinople. Ever since the Edict of Thessalonica in 380 (which formally made Christianity the state religion), the Empire was officially Christian. And the Christian veterinarians of Byzantium were important enough in shaping veterinary medicine that their influence lasted for over half a millennium.

Byzantine veterinarians were pioneers in the area of equine medicine particularly. Hierokles' statement that "the horse is considered to be the most beautiful animal, and the most precious to mankind"[iii] may give us an idea of the prime importance of the equid species in Byzantine society. Nearly all the writings from Byzantine veterinarians deal with horses. Throughout the Middle Ages they were republished and still relied upon as late as the 16th century.

There were Byzantium agricultural works, such as *The Geoponica*, which included sections on animal medicine. But it was a massive text on the treatment of diseases and injuries of horses called the *Corpus Hippiatricorum Graecorpum* (a title mercifully shortened to *Hippiatrika*) that became the major contribution of Byzantine Christians to the developing field of veterinary medicine. This massive work collected the writings of 17 Byzantine veterinarians and covered treatments for a host of conditions including lameness, trauma (particularly related to wounds suffered by war horses), dystocia, nutrition, digestive diseases, and contagious diseases.

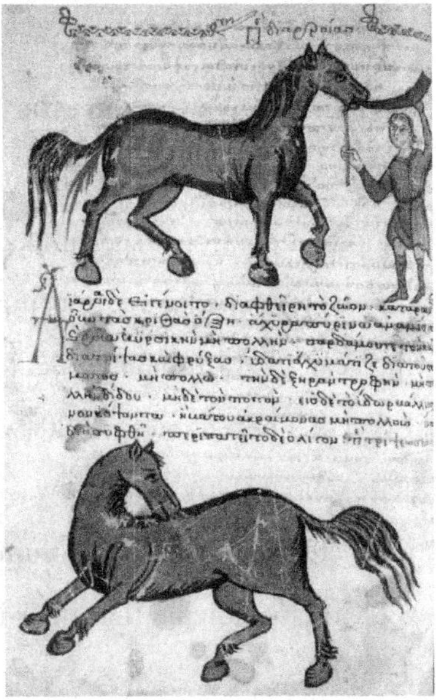

Illustration demonstrating the drenching of a horse for diarrhea, from a 14th century folio edition of the Hippiatrika.

Apsyrtos, Emperor Constantine's military veterinarian, was prominent among the contributors to the *Hippiatrika*.

His writing incorporated the medical reasoning of Hippocrates, the theoretical medical teachings of ancient writers, and his own practical experience in treating army horses. This amazing Greek was born in Asia Minor in 300 AD. Unfortunately, we know little about his life. We find an intriguing entry in the *Souda*, the universal lexicon of the Empire, which describes Apsyrtos as "a soldier" and states he "was on campaign under the Emperor Constantine, in Scythia along the river Danube."[iv] This is probably a reference to Constantine's campaigns against the Goths and the Samaritans in 332 and 334. It seems likely the armies of New Rome had a corps of veterinarians much like the human medical corps we know existed. The work of Apsyrtos as the chief veterinarian for the army would likely have entailed the training and oversight of all the other veterinarians in this body. He may have also served a sort of consulting role, giving advice and lending equipment to soldiers, who normally looked after their own horses.[v] Apsyrtos made one hundred and twenty-one contributions to the corpus of the *Hipiatrika*, all as letters to his colleagues. His works directly affected many other contributors to the *Hipiatrika*, and he is considered one of the most influential and prominent of ancient veterinary writers.

We can imagine Apsyrtos as an adventurer and soldier, a noted thinker and teacher, and a member of the top echelon of early Byzantine society. A typical day in his profession might have included shouting instructions to aides above the roar of battle, while surgically extracting an arrow from some great general's fallen horse (a surgery in which he would have used an ingenious device known as the "spoon of Diokles" to minimize tissue trauma). A typical day might also have brought him into counsel with the Emperor to answer questions about his favorite horse or advise him about the soundness of a particular racing steed at the hippodrome (chariot racing and a type of polo formed very popular diversions for all classes of Byzantine society). It would be no stretch of the imagination to consider his spare time consumed with reading the latest texts of medical theorists. He probably explored animal anatomy and physiology, trying to advance the knowledge of a practice denigrated for centuries.

The Horse

The extensive use of horses in transport, agriculture, and military conquest made them the dominant species of interest to veterinarians from ancient times well into the 18th century. Earlier veterinarians were often viewed as "blue-collar" mechanics for horses throughout the Middle Ages, and farriers (horseshoers) were viewed as the experts in veterinary medicine in the early modern era, before the development of veterinary schools and the dawn of professional veterinary medicine.

There were other contributors to the veterinary text we know as the *Hippiatrika.* Heirokles worked as a lawyer in 350 AD but was interested in equine medicine enough to write about it. He contributed 107 entries to the *Hippiatrika* and may have been the author (under a pseudonym) of another ten-volume book on equine medicine called the *Mulomedicina Chironis.* A man named Publius Vegetius Renatus also contributed to the *Hippiatrika* and wrote another work of his own on veterinary medicine, the *Artis Veterinariae, Sive Mulomedicinae.* We don't know a lot about Vegetius, as he is more commonly called, but suspect he was a Byzantine nobleman interested in veterinary medicine. He wrote about livestock as well as horses.

The authors of the *Hippiatrika* were likely in a higher social status than the average veterinarian. In his prologues to the *Mulomedicinae*, Vegetius bemoaned the state of the Byzantine veterinary profession, complaining it paid very little and was considered a lowly occupation. Much is speculative when dealing with history so ancient. But it seems likely they viewed veterinarians as "blue-collar" workers, which is a situation we'll find throughout the early stages of the profession.

Nevertheless, it appears evident an average Byzantine veterinarian was at least literate—most of the veterinary writings were addressed to them. These writings also indicate the specialized veterinarian understood anatomy and physiology. He possibly employed a technical language unique to his profession (in addition to terminology shared by human physicians), analogous to the technical language we use in the profession today.

Dunlop and Williams (in their seminal work *Veterinary Medicine, an Illustrated History*) call the Byzantine veterinarians "trailblazers who succeeded in raising veterinary clinical competence to a high level, especially in equine medicine. They created a focus on veterinary diagnostic, therapeutic, and preventative medicine with a moderate and rational basis."[vi] And they grew out of the Christian cultural landscape of the Byzantine Empire.

Other Medieval Cultures

Even in the Arab world, which played its own significant role in the development of veterinary medicine, Christians worked to advance theoretical and clinical aspects of animal health.

Nestorian Christians played an important role in translating Greek writings for the scholarly Umayyad Caliphate during a revival of learning in the Arab domain. This included writings of influential medical works and promoted thinking about medical theory. It was a Christian apothecary family in Iraq who produced Hunayn, a writer with veterinary interests who translated the veterinary writings of Theomnestus into Arabic and pioneered work in the field of ophthalmology.

In medieval Europe, veterinary medicine was slower to develop and would seem deplorable by modern medical standards. Veterinarians were usually called "ox-leeches" or "horse-leeches" and wrote treatises based on their experience along with scraps gleaned from ancient writers. They were not respectable members of society. Much of their work was not medicine at all but relied on charms and amulets based on the superstition originating from pagan traditions, blended with a Roman Catholic fascination of miracles. Herbal remedies (oral mixtures and topical poultices) were used as well. Unfortunately, treatment of animal disease in medieval Europe could be cruel, and worse than the disease itself. This was equally true of human medicine.

But significantly, medieval Christians cared enough to practice medicine on animals at all. Though they are sparse, some medical writings were preserved, read, and practiced during the "dark ages" of medieval Europe.

Along with the revivals of learning in the 14th and 15th centuries came discoveries and methodology in veterinary medicine in many Christian countries of Europe. One example is *Libro de Albeyteria por lo Noble Mossen Manuel Diaz*, a significant work on equine medicine written by Marshall Don Manuel Diaz in 1443. This book collected veterinary information learned in a war campaign in Naples, commissioned by Alphonse V, King of Spain, an ardent patron of veterinary medicine. Another Spaniard, Don Juan Suarez de Peralta, wrote the first known veterinary work in the new world in 1580.

During the late Medieval Era, laws were passed to improve veterinary standards among some westerners. A prime example was in Spain, where Christian rulers Isabel and Ferdinand improved on Moorish albeytar system of equine medicine (a way of practicing

---

"Many of the early giants in the advancement of medical knowledge were devoted Christians and motivated by Christian ideals."

---

and teaching horse medicine) by adding a regulatory body (the "protoalbeytars").

Christians Who Advanced Medical Theory

Veterinary medical theory (as opposed to practice) developed along with human medicine, through the study of comparative anatomy and physiology. Indeed, it often played a pivotal role in advancing human medicine, since animal models were used to study anatomy and physiology. And many of the early giants in the advancement of medical knowledge were devoted Christians and motivated by Christian ideals.

Following are a few examples, meant to be representative rather than exhaustive, of researchers whose Christian faith influenced their work, and whose work, in turn, influenced both human and veterinary medicine.

- **Henri de Mondeville** (1260-1320), a Parisian surgeon, advanced the practice of surgery by basing it soundly on physiology, introducing tourniquets and ligation, and arguing for sanitary practices and surgical prep of wounds. In his book *La Chirurgia* he argued God heals through the efforts of skilled surgeons more often than He does through miracles alone.
- **Paracelsus** (1493-1541), whose actual name was Theophrastus von Hohenheim. No wonder he went by Paracelsus! This giant of medical theory challenged the Renaissance

tradition of relying on only a few favored classical writers on which to base medical theory, in favor of medicine based on experimentation and science. He once dramatically threw a copy of *Cannon of Medicine* by Avicenna into a bonfire to symbolize the need for revival in medical thinking. He was instrumental in the development of toxicology, and is famous for saying "dose alone makes the poison."[vii] Though tainted by astrology and occultist ideas, the philosophies of Paracelsus were grounded in a Christian belief in God. He once wrote that "God, our Father, has given us the life and the art of healing to protect and maintain it."[viii]

Valerius Cordus (1515-1544) advanced evidence-based pharmacology with his edit of *Dispensatorium Pharmacopolarum* in 1535. He also is credited with the invention of ether, which became widely used for early anesthesia. Cordus was an ardent Lutheran and an intellectual product of the Protestant Reformation.

Ambrose Paré (1510-1590) was "the greatest figure in the history of surgery in the sixteenth century."[ix] The son of a poor cabinetmaker, he started his career as an apprentice to a barber surgeon—who were despised as low class, callous, and barbaric. But he developed and refined the field of surgery with his remarkable skills as a surgeon (it was said he could perform an amputation in three minutes). He was a scientist and accomplished controlled studies in wound healing. He wrote many books, one of which (*La Méthode de Traiter les*

Playes Faites par Hacquebutes V. 2) was devoted to veterinary surgery. Paré once said that““the surgeon dressed wounds but God healed them””[x] Paré's compassion for his patients and concern for relieving both human and animal suffering made him stand out in a harsh age.

Robert Boyle (1627-1692) established that animal bodies need an element in the air to survive (oxygen), and was a forerunner in the concept and study of blood gasses. He was a devoted Christian who wrote that scientific research is a way man can grow closer to God. Robert Hooke, Boyle's lab assistant, demonstrated that artificial respiration could keep a dog alive. Hooke also contributed research to the theory that led to the development of the microscope.

Michael Harward practiced livestock medicine in England and Ireland in the 17th century. He condemned many of the superstitious practices of the "ox-leeches" in his book *The Herdsman's Mate*, published in 1673. He described many animal diseases and treatments (including 17th century neurosurgery descriptions), and encouraged others to practice thoughtful medicine "blessed by God."[xi] He was particularly influential in developing veterinary methods of abdominal surgery and described in amazing accuracy end-to-end resection and anastomosis in cattle many years before any human surgeon.

Francesco Redi (1626-1697), the father of parasitology, studied and wrote extensively about parasites infesting animals. He was a Christian and originally trained by Catholic Jesuits. He once drank snake venom to prove that it had to be injected to affect a victim!

- **Bernardino Ramazzini** (1633-1714) was educated by Jesuits and went on to study medicine and philosophy in Padua. He wrote an early and excellent work describing rinderpest disease in cattle and invented a type of early vaccination. His work in epidemiology has led to him being called its founder. He also became an early expert on occupational diseases.
- **Stephen Hales** (1677-1761) was an English preacher and self-taught scientist. He pioneered research in physiology, making a particular impact in fluid dynamics. He performed a famous experiment to measure the blood pressure and pulse rate of a horse.
- **Albrecht von Haller** (1708-1777), called "the father of modern physiology," wrote about the functional aspect of animal bodies. He was active in building the Reformed Church in Gottingen, Germany, and wrote Christian texts.
- **Johan Göze** (1731-1793) pioneered work on helminthology (gastrointestinal worms) and published an influential book on parasitology in animals in 1787 (*Versuch einer Naturgeschichte der Eingeweidewürmer tierischer Körper*). He was an amateur naturalist, but also studied theology at the University of Halle and was a German pastor. He became the first deacon of the seminary of Quedlinburg.
- **Lazzaro Spallanzani** (1729-1799) was a brilliant medical

researcher and professor in Modeno and Pavia and an ordained priest in Italy (sometimes called Abbe or Abbate). He did important work in digestion and cardiac physiology, as well as research to refute the still-popular idea of spontaneous generation (the theory that animals can evolve from non-living compounds). Abbe Lazzaro researched animal medicine and was the first scientist to successfully perform artificial insemination on a dog and proved that sperm is necessary for fertilization.

Dr. Benjamin Rush (1746-1813) was a founding father of the United States, a signer of the Declaration of Independence, and a brilliant physician. He was also an outspoken Christian, in charge of America's first Bible Society. In 1807 Rush wrote a call for veterinary education, which helped promote New World awareness of the developing veterinary profession in Europe.

Gregor Mendel (1822-1884) is the father of modern genetics and made breakthroughs in our understanding of inheritance. His work affects many aspects of veterinary medicine, from understanding congenital diseases to animal breeding and theriogenology. He was also an Augustinian monk who lived and worked at the Monastery of St. Thomas in Brno, Moravia.

Charles Barkla (1877-1944) opened the way for using x-rays to take radiographs. He was a devout Methodist who sought God through science.

- **John Eccles** (1903-1997) performed groundbreaking research to describe the synapse of neurons (where one nerve connects to another) which won a Nobel Prize. He was a Catholic who professed belief in God's work over nature.
- **Francis Collins** (1950-present) invented cloning. He was originally an atheist who came to Christ.

These men all advanced our understanding of medical theory, some in animal medicine primarily, and some in human medicine. And what is significant to the point of this study, every one of them came from an intellectual background of Christian faith. Many were outspoken about the way their faith influenced their scientific work.

"Though professional veterinary education may have had roots in the French Enlightenment culture, those very roots were planted in a Christian soil, and reached down deep through the ages of Christian tradition."

Birth of the Veterinary Profession in France

It was in the 18th century that veterinary medicine began to stand on its own as a distinct profession and gained respectability along with its human counterpart. This was largely due to the advent of true veterinary education.

The very first school exclusively devoted to training veterinarians was commissioned in Lyon, France on August 4, 1761. It is significant that (out of all the places in the world this might have happened) it was a Christian country, under the influence of a Christian culture, which produced men who deemed animal health important enough to open a school devoted to its teaching. The school in Lyon sparked a veterinary revolution throughout the west, and by 1800 19 new veterinary schools opened across Christian countries of Europe. This is not a coincidence. Christians had been heavily involved in advancing medical research in the preceding centuries and had strong theological motivation to follow Christ in pushing back the front lines of suffering in the war on disease in both humans and animals.

France at this time was in the throes of the "enlightenment," a time when new ideas in science and philosophy bloomed. Many of these ideas challenged blind faith in traditions based on classical authors (in science and medicine) or teachings of the church (in philosophy). A group of scholars called "le Encyclopédistes" (the encyclopedists) played a pivotal role in this intellectual revolution. This group of over 150 scholars boasted famous historical figures such as Denis Diderot, Charles Montesquieu, and Jean-Jacques Rousseau. It also included Charles Bourgelat, history's first director of a veterinary school.

Enlightenment scholars, sometimes called "renaissance humanists," espoused a humanism that was sometimes less a celebration of humanity's knowledge than it was a reactionary anti-Christian philosophy. French scholars date the Enlightenment in their country from 1715 to 1789. It ended in the bloodbaths of the French revolution, which was in many ways the political child birthed of Enlightenment philosophy.

The veterinary school near Lyon opened its doors in 1762, at a building called the Inn of the Abundance. The first class comprised 38 students, one of whom was only 11 years old! There were no age requirements for applying to the school, though the ability to read and write was mandatory. Interestingly, there was also a requirement that students present a record of baptism.[xii] This is a reminder that, though professional veterinary education may have had roots in French Enlightenment culture, those very Enlightenment roots were planted in Christian soil, and reached down deep through ages of Christian tradition. The French Royal Controller-General of Agriculture, Henri-Leonard-Jean Baptist Bertin, commissioned his friend Claude Bourgelat as the school's first director in 1761.

The first curriculum of the school at Lyon was largely focused on the horse. But, probably because of Bertin's influence, livestock medicine was also studied. Students followed a model of instruction centered on copying and reciting verbatim the lessons of Director Bourgelat. But

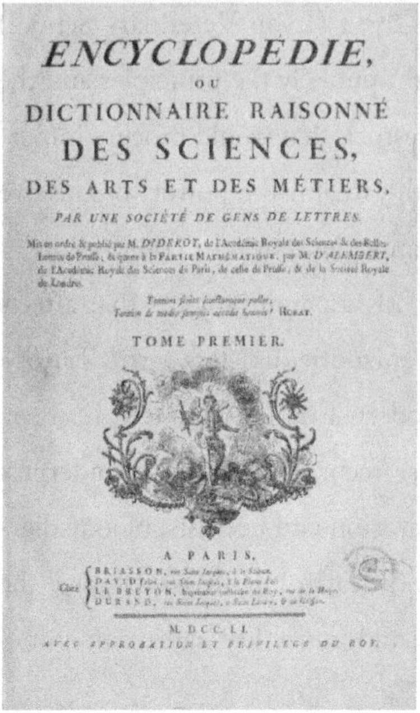
ENCYCLOPÉDIE,
OU
DICTIONNAIRE RAISONNÉ
DES SCIENCES,
DES ARTS ET DES MÉTIERS,
PAR UNE SOCIÉTÉ DE GENS DE LETTRES.
Mis en ordre & publié par M. DIDEROT, de l'Académie Royale des Sciences & des Belles-Lettres de Prusse; & quant à la PARTIE MATHÉMATIQUE, par M. D'ALEMBERT, de l'Académie Royale des Sciences de Paris, de celle de Prusse, & de la Société Royale de Londres.
TOME PREMIER.
A PARIS,
Chez BRIASSON, DAVID, LE BRETON, DURAND
M. DCC. LI.
AVEC APPROBATION ET PRIVILEGE DU ROY.

"Encyclopedia, or a Systemic Dictionary of the Sciences, Arts, and Crafts" was the work and raison d'etre (reason of being) of the French Encylopedists. The finished product consisted of 17 volumes of text and 11 volumes of pictures, purporting to be a summary of mankind's knowledge in its entirety. There is not, at this time, a graphic novel edition.

their education was not limited to lessons on paper, and they took part in demonstrations on dissection and botany (in the "herbarium") and practiced medicine and animal care under the direct supervision of teachers.

There were three "theoretical courses" students were required to take in those early years of the school. "The first was devoted to the study of external parts, animal osteology, and mycology. The second was devoted to 'materia medica,' splanchnology, and bandaging. The third was devoted to physiology, medicine, pharmacology, and the appropriate use of medications."[xiii]

King Louis XV invested heavily in the new school, giving a grant of 50,000 livres (roughly 540 ounces of gold). He was concerned about the state of agriculture in his country, especially regarding the livestock disease called rinderpest. The Royal decree installing L'Ecole Vétérinaire de Lyon (Lyon Veterinary School) read that students would be "taught publicly the principles and the method to cure the diseases of livestock that would procure imperceptibly from the agriculture of the Realm the power to conserve livestock in times where this epidemic desolates the countryside."[xiv]

Rinderpest (or "cattle plague") is a paramyxovirus that affects ruminants and raged in multiple epizootic disasters across Europe from the Middle Ages to the Modern Era. (Fortunately, it's been eradicated, the last confirmed case recorded in 2001.) Rinderpest virus caused fever, anorexia, oral erosion and necrosis, bloody diarrhea, dehydration, emaciation, and death. Highly contagious, the morbidity rate was near 100% and mortality rates sometimes reached 90%. It killed millions of animals, contributed to human starvation, and crippled the economy of affected countries. It should be no surprise that researching methods for controlling rinderpest were a major motivation in the development of early veterinary medicine.

The massive impact of rinderpest on human and animal suffering made it something the church had to address more than once. One good example occurred in the early 18th century when the Catholic Church took an active interest in a panzootic episode of rinderpest under the guidance of Giovanni Mario Lancisi (1654-1720), who was the court physician of the Pope. After investigating an outbreak of herd disease, he found it to be rinderpest that had spread from Russia through Sweden to the rest of Europe. He convinced the College of Cardinals there was no cure and they should slaughter all affected livestock to prevent the outbreak from spreading. This drastic measure rendered the region of Padua free of rinderpest in nine months.

In contrast, it spread through the rest of Europe for years (killing over two hundred million cattle)[xv] and caused devastating problems for these countries' economies, including France.

The new school bore fruit, and in recognition of the school's research and fieldwork (especially regarding rinderpest), King Louis granted the title "Royale" to the school. L'Ecole Vétérinaire Royale de Lyon pushed forward the boundaries of medical knowledge and made significant strides in fighting epizootic diseases through its research over the years.

In 1793 (while the Reign of Terror raged across France) the school's director saved the students and animals during a bombardment that destroyed its facility by moving them to his lands at Eailly. In 1796 the school relocated to the Cloitre de Deux Amants, an ancient French convent. The school ended up trained many of the early giants in the formation of the new profession of veterinary medicine.

Claude Bourgelat (1712-1779), the first director of a veterinary school, was a fascinating man whom we might imagine in the image of Cyrano de Bergerac. Claude was the product of a turbulent and epic era. Unfortunately (yet again, much like the fictitious Cyrano), Claude had a reputation as a vain and often argumentative fellow. But his skills as a leader and his knowledge of equine medicine providentially positioned him at the right moment to organize the center of the modern profession of veterinary medicine.

He was born into French aristocracy and studied law. But he became disenchanted with the legal profession after he saw his work help free a guilty man and joined the army. The cavalryman was a vital part of France's military and horsemanship a paramount skill—one in which Bourgelat excelled. He became famous

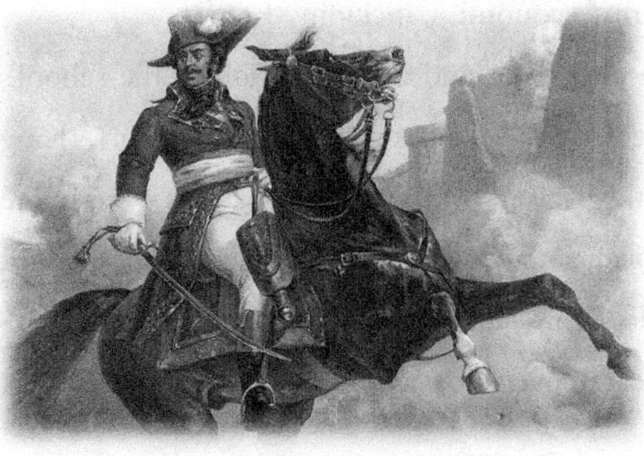

This oil painting of Général Alexandre Dumas by Olivier Pichat [US-PD] is a good representation of the French cavalry.

enough for his equestrian ability and knowledge that Austrian Emperor Frederick the Great even consulted him on horsemanship. Bourgelat eventually left the army and became master of the Lyon Academy of Equitation, where he taught the sons of noblemen the arts of horsemanship, saber fighting, and chivalry. Chivalry had certainly degraded by Claude's day from its roots as a robust and Christian warrior code to become more of a fashionable list of rules for polite society: but it would have retained some of the creeds of its long Christian heritage.

While he taught at the Academy, Bourgelat spent time under the guidance of two surgeons in Lyon, studying medicine to improve his understanding of veterinary medicine. Bourgelat's veterinary studies, his connections with French nobility (especially Bertin), and his chivalrous training made him an ideal head of the new veterinary school. Bourgelat later headed another veterinary school founded in Paris in 1765. Soon thereafter this school moved to an impressive castle, Le Chateau d'Alfort, and Bourgelat's title was upgraded to "Inspector-General of all Veterinary Schools."

Later **Etienne Guillaume LaFosse, Sr.** (1738-1820) of Montataire started a rival, private veterinary school. He spent much of his career vilifying and arguing with Bourgelat. He was an early pioneer of veterinary medicine who helped raise equine medicine to a professional level based on sound scientific and medical knowledge. His work on equine lameness with its colored illustrations was especially influential. He advocated major changes in the shoeing practices of his day which would improve equine health and comfort. His son Philippe-Etienne LaFosse, Jr. expanded his father's work.

Spreading like wildfire from France, the idea of an elevated, more scientific profession of veterinary medicine grew under the influence of more than one Christian nation.

Dutch Influence

An influential professor: **Hermann Boerhaave** (1688-1738) was a Dutch physician, professor (of medicine, and botany, and chemistry), and "arguably the greatest medical thinker of the eighteenth century."[xvi] He has been called the "Dutch Hippocrates." Hermann Boerhaave's greatest legacy is his many students found among the ranks of veterinary medicine's founders.

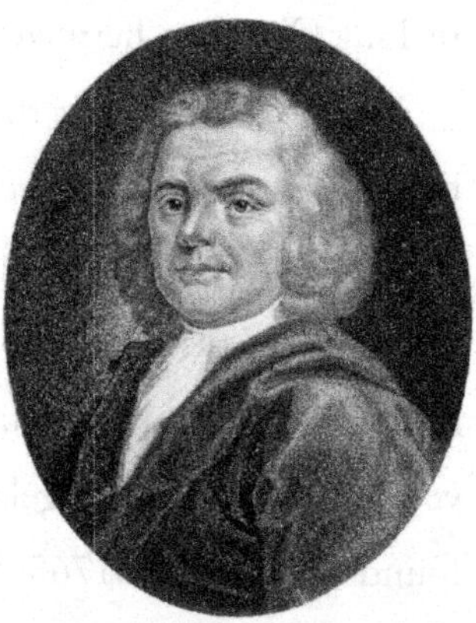

Hermann Boerhaave, in a 1798 portrait by J. Chapman

He was the son of a Reformed minister, in a time not far removed from the advent of Protestantism in Holland—the first Dutch Protestant synod was in 1571. Perhaps it should be no surprise that Boerhaave originally wanted to study theology and become a preacher like his father. Contemporaries report his faith was more than academic or culturally motivated, but deeply personal. One of Boerhaave's biographers wrote that he "experienced a secret intercourse with God. However heavy were his tasks for the day, each morning he spent an hour in prayer and meditations."[xvii]

He studied philosophy on a scholarship at the University of Leiden. *De distinctione mentis a corpore* (on the distinction between mind and body) was the title of his thesis. He went on to study medicine and became a physician in 1693. He never left the University of Leiden and spent the next 36 years teaching botany, medicine, and chemistry. Boerhaave rejected the superstitions and dogmatic assumptions of many of his forebears and espoused a rigorously scientific method of medicine instead.

Boerhaave was most influential through his teaching—though he made significant advancements in medical practice as well (such as discovering the compound urea and introducing the thermometer to medical practice).

His clinical method of teaching, grounded in a compassionate bedside manner, revolutionized the way medicine was taught. It also attracted a slew of disciples who became influential in the development of modern veterinary and human medicine.

Austro-Hungarian Influence

Gerard van Swieten (1700-1772) was the chief medical officer of the Austro-Hungarian Empire, and Empress Maria-Theresa's favorite counselor and personal physician. He had a direct influence on the development of veterinary medicine in his country through his efforts to organize it from his government office as a respected discipline.

Born into a Dutch family from Leiden and an orphan at 12,

around the time he graduated from Latin School. He originally studied philosophy at Leiden University, before changing his mind to study pharmacology. He spent five years as a pharmacist in Leiden and studied medicine (under Herman Boerhaave for much of the time). Van Swieten became a physician in 1725, studying under Boerhaave for the next 13 years—he's said to have only missed one of Boerhaave's lectures the entire time! Besides practicing, van Swieten taught medicine until 1734. He married Maria Beeck van Coesfelt in 1729 and had six children over the years of their reportedly happy union. One of his sons, Godfried, became an Austrian ambassador and a notable patron of music (supporting Mozart, Hayden, and Beethoven in particular).

In 1745, van Swieten moved his family to Vienna to become Empress Maria-Theresa's court physician. She was famous for her Catholic devotion (as well as her intolerant views toward Protestants and Jews) and sought van Swieten since he was a Dutch Catholic. Van Swieten's Catholicism is worth noting, given his cultural setting in Leiden, which was not far removed from the Dutch civil war (The Eighty Years' War) that had resulted in a strict (anti-Catholic) Calvinism being declared the state religion under William of Orange. He would have been in the religious minority. Jesuits (famous for their religious zeal) had baptized him. These factors make it likely van Swieten's faith was more than just familial or cultural: he had much to lose by it.

As chief medical officer in Austria, van Swieten worked exhaustively to build a more modern, evidence-based medicine. In addition to reforming human medical education, he consciously worked to build a system of education in veterinary medicine. He envisioned the two disciplines working in tandem, with similar principles of comparative anatomy, elevating both to professional levels. He wanted to start a school. Had the time been right van Swieten might have shaped veterinary medicine into something loftier than the "animal mechanic" job it was limited to in his country.

After consulting veterinarians from the school in Lyon, van Swieten realized more scientific and detailed studies in animal disease needed to be performed before establishing modern veterinary education. He decided eradication of rinderpest (which moved largely over trade routes passing through Austro-Hungary) was a more pressing concern than establishing new veterinary schools.

Van Swieten commissioned a Slovakian colleague, **Pál Adámi** (1739-1814), to study veterinary medicine with this goal in mind. He tasked Adámi to do exhaustive veterinary field research, learn animal medicine, and then lead a revolution of veterinary training in the Austro-Hungarian Empire. Adámi was another student of Hermann Boerhaave. He wrote extensively on veterinary diseases, their prevention, and their cures. He did brilliant work and developed inoculation methods for several diseases, including rinderpest and foot and mouth disease (using thread inoculated with diseased saliva that was attenuated by air drying). He became influential in epidemiology, and the empress appointed him as professor of medicine and epizootiology at the University of Vienna. Unfortunately,

Adámi rose and fell with the political machinations of his friends—he lost his job after Maria-Theresa's death. Eventually, he became the professor of veterinary medicine at the school in Krakow in 1804.

One of Adámi's pupils, **A.A. Rudnicki,** followed in his steps to become the first Polish veterinary professor. The first official Polish veterinary school, the Institute for Veterinary Medicine in Rzadowa, opened in 1840, and Poland would go on to develop a rich tradition of veterinary medicine in its own right.

After Maria-Theresa's death, her son Joseph II took an interest in veterinary medicine from a practical, militaristic standpoint. The Austrian emperor visited Bourgelat's Paris school at le Chateaux d'Alfort in 1777, which confirmed his desire for a local school producing competent equine veterinarians. In 1769, on the advice of his councilors, he commissioned an army field doctor named **Johann Gottlieb Wolstein** (1738-1820) to study veterinary medicine, intending to start a new school and bring leadership to Austria's veterinarians. Wolstein studied at the Paris school initially, but he soon went over to the private school of LaFosse, Jr. (with whom he developed a friendship that would last his lifetime). Later he toured the British Isles to learn more about ovine (sheep) and equine care and studied in Holland and Germany

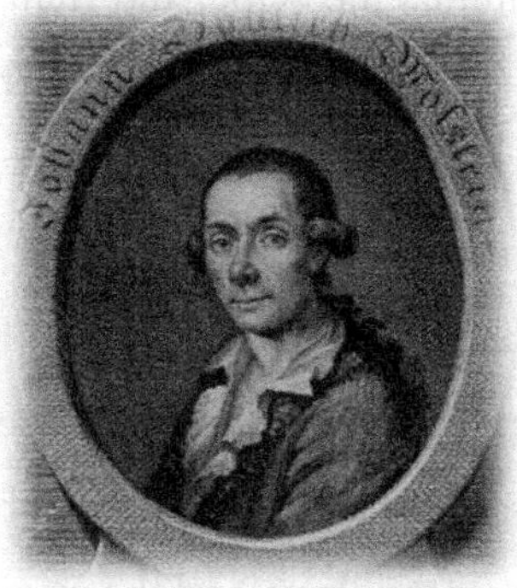

Stipple engraving of Johann Gottlieb Wolstein

and Denmark. He finally obtained a surgeon's degree in Jena in 1775.

Wolstein designed an improved veterinary school upon his return to Vienna. He also established a Hungarian veterinary school in Budapest. Wolstein condemned the negligent and unhygienic livestock practices of his day. He erroneously argued it was lack of sanitation and quality care, not contagion, which caused rinderpest.

Wolstein was a Protestant Christian persecuted for his faith, with religious convictions that ended in his arrest in 1794 by Catholic authorities. They also persecuted him for expressing "Jacobin" sentiments, extreme republican revolutionary ideas associated with the French revolution. He eventually escaped prison but had to flee the country. He lived out his remaining 25 years of life in Germany.

German Influence

By the time Wolstein fled to Germany, it was developing a veterinary profession of its own, under the leadership of the brilliant and charismatic **Johann Christian Polycarp Erxleben** (1744-1777).

"He [Erxleben] had connections with the local church, and enlisted priests to tell their parishioners about his new veterinary program to bring in patients."

Johann's father was a deacon of Quedlinburg and a poor man with a large family. His remarkable mother, Dorothea Christine

Erxleben, was the first woman to study at a German University. Family difficulties interrupted her studies when her brother dodged a draft, causing her father to desert the family. Dorothea stayed home to provide for them through her medical work until her marriage at 27. After a prolonged course of study, she graduated from medical school at Halle in 1754.

It was Johann Erxleben who first proposed a veterinary course at the University of Göttingen in an unsolicited letter to the university curator in 1768. This was a brazen move! He was only 24 years old at the time and had never finished his medical degree (though he had studied chemistry and medicine). He asked the government to create a veterinary school and let him teach in it. What's more, he presented in the letter a detailed plan for his professorship. This was a daring proposal in a time when veterinary medicine in Germany was not considered important enough to be taught in a university. The 80-year-old King GA von Munchausen approved the plan, just three days after reading the letter, and also asked Erxleben to write a book. In 1769 Johann published *Introduction to Veterinary Medicine.* The king sent Erxleben to study more formally at Cologne (with von Sind), in Holland, and at Lyon until 1770.

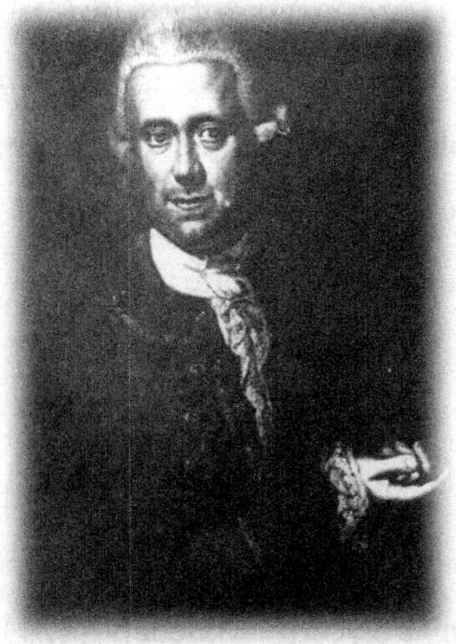

Johann Christian Polycarp Erxleben

He returned to become the first German professor of veterinary medicine, teaching tirelessly at the brand-new vet school at the University of Göttingen. He was also a member of the philosophy faculty. He treated local animals for free two days per week to provide clinical experience for his students. He had connections with the local church and enlisted priests to tell their parishioners about his new veterinary program to bring in patients. The veterinary program was a two-year course, and it required students to be at least 18 years old and know both Latin and French.

Sadly, Erxleben died early at age 34. A veterinary school established in Hannover in 1778 eventually superseded the school at Göttingen. But it was Erxleben's remarkable efforts that started the profession on its useful course in Germany.

Another influential German was **Baron J.B. von Sind** (1709-1776), who Johann trained with for a time. Von Sind was a German cavalry officer, an expert on equine care, and an early advocate for the humane treatment of animal patients (specifically condemning the cruel practices common among farriers in his day). Von Sind wrote *Introduction to the Science of the Stallmeister*, which presented many medical innovations, including improved methods of surgical restraints and better ways to treat fractures.

Scottish Influence

James Clark (1732-1808) of Edinburgh, Scotland was an early veterinary practitioner and writer, who labored to improve the humane treatment of animal patients. He was extremely well-read and educated and known for his compassion and concern for his animal patients in a time in Scotland when medical treatment could hurt worse than the disease. He published three books on veterinary medicine. He described many diseases accurately and with practical and conservative treatments, based more on observation of clinical signs and contemporary medical theory than medieval folk remedies or humoral theory of the horse-leech. He devoted an entire chapter of his book *Treatise on the Prevention of Disease (Incidental to Horses)* to kindness toward horses.

James Clark called attention to the lack of a veterinary school in Scotland and wanted one started in Edinburgh. Though he would not see this dream become a reality in his life, shortly afterward **William Dick** (1793-1866) started the Dick School of Veterinary Medicine in Edinburgh in 1833. The school is still in operation today. Several veterinarians who studied there established an important school in Canada, which influenced veterinary medicine in the United States. North American veterinarians can thank William Dick for his indirect influence on bringing professional veterinary medicine to the New World.

"There I admire the wisdom of the Creator, which manifests itself in so many various modes, and demonstrate it to others."
– Carl Linnaeus to the University of Uppsala

Swedish Influence

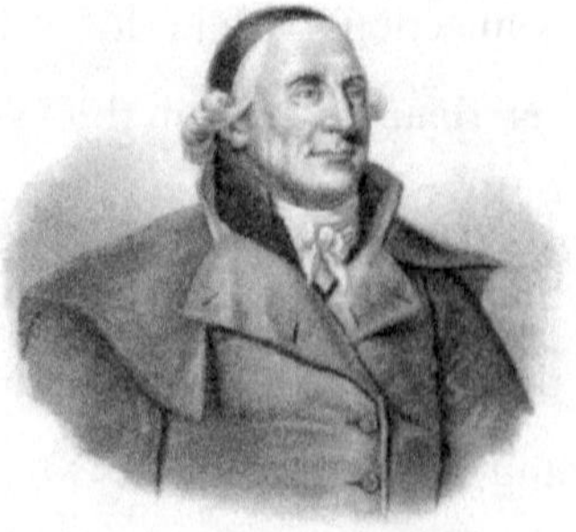

Peter Hernquist

Peter Hernquist (1726-1808) was a student of the brilliant zoologist and physician Carl Linnaeus[xviii] in Sweden. He studied at Uppsala University, mastering in philosophy at Greifswald University. Declining an offer to teach botany at St. Petersburg, Hernquist went to France and studied veterinary medicine at Bourgelat's new school from 1763 to 1766. He stayed in Paris teaching for a while and built a botanical garden for the city (the Jardin des Plantes).

Hernquist returned to Sweden when his country's government contacted him with a commission to start a new veterinary school in 1769. But government funding was postponed, and he spent the next few years teaching mathematics at Skara while he worked on planning the school. At last, in 1775 the funding came through for an official veterinary school. The builders discovered a medieval monastery as the foundation was dug, delaying construction of the new school building. Hernquist took a break to supervise the archaeological excavation. When the school was finally built, Hernquist taught while he practiced as a physician on both humans and animals. He was particularly interested in broadening the scope of veterinary medicine beyond its current equine focus and did important work with livestock.

A colorful, well-rounded scholar, Hernquist maintained a veterinary museum on campus. Like Erxleben, Hernquist utilized connections with his local church to help improve the reputation of veterinary science, in this case through music. He required students to have a good singing voice and started a veterinary school choir that sang at the local church. He planted three trees he named after the founders of modern veterinary medicine (Bourgelat, LaFosse, and Abildgaard). His 30 years of work at the school raised the standards and reputation of the modern profession of veterinary medicine. His work is continued by the Swedish University of Agricultural Sciences in Skara today and commemorated at the Veterinary Museum at Brogården (where one can also visit the 13th century Franciscan monastery of St. Catherine that Hernquist excavated).

Denmark Influence

Peter Christian Abildgaard (1740-1801) was a Danish student sent by his government to Lyon to study veterinary medicine in 1763. He, like Hernquist, became disappointed in the new profession's obsession with equine medicine. An apt scholar, Abildgaard finished the three-year course in only two years and found it necessary to supplement deficiencies in teaching on internal medicine with his own studies of human medicine and comparative anatomy. He obtained a medical degree in 1768.

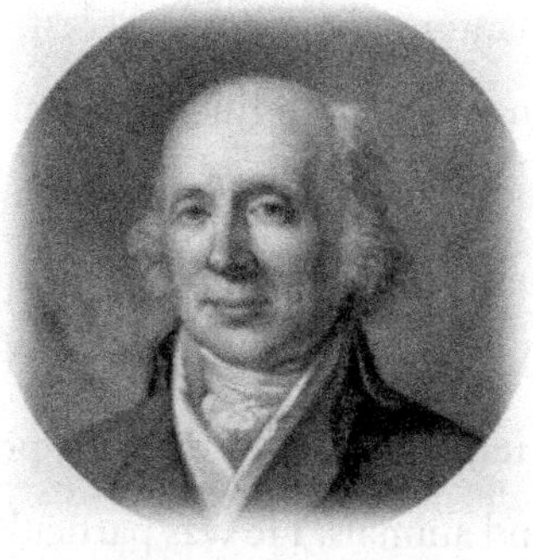

Peter Christian Abildgaard

He eventually headed a new veterinary school in Copenhagen, approved (but only partially funded) by the government in 1773. In 1777 his school became a public institution, fully funded by the government. He worked out a system with the government for recruiting students from Denmark and Normandy to improve agriculture. They recruited a literate son of a blacksmith or farmer every three years and subsidized the cost of his education at Abildgaard's school—with the proviso the man would return to his diocese and practice on livestock there. Abildgaard also devised an eradication protocol for rinderpest. A diverse scholar, he had a personal library of 2156 books, only about 10% of which were in veterinary medicine. His diverse interests included medicine, zoology, physics (he even built a hot-air balloon), economics, politics, and geology.

"I am convinced there is no part of India where the pure religion of the Gospel might be introduced with a fairer prospect of success."
– William Moorcroft, writing about Kashmir

English Influence

William Moorcroft (1767-1825) was a veterinarian, explorer, and possibly a British spy. History provides William Moorcroft to reassure anyone who doubts a veterinarian can be an adventurer too! Moorcroft was England's first officially trained veterinarian, ran a booming equine practice in London for many years, and contributed to veterinary knowledge (especially in equine lameness).

He was the illegitimate son of a prominent dairyman's daughter in Ormskirk, Lancashire. He lived with his grandfather Richard, read from his extensive library, and learned riding and agricultural practices on his farm. A neighbor, Thomas Eccleston, took an interest in Moorcroft. William called him "my more than father." Eccleston was known across England for his progressive farming methods, and he passed his fascination with agricultural technology to young William. When it was time for Moorcroft to find a trade, he went to Liverpool to apprentice as a surgeon under Dr. John Lyon (probably through connections of Eccleston, who contributed funds to the infirmary there). Moorcroft did so well in his studies that, in 1786, he was offered both a job in the hospital and a partnership in Lyon's practice. It was a promising start to a career in human surgery.

But his career took an unexpected turn when Thomas Eccleston sent to the Liverpool Infirmary for help with a sudden cattle plague decimating his herds. William came back to the farm but was frustrated he could do nothing more than have the carcasses buried to prevent further disease from spreading. In the end, this became the impetus for Moorcroft's decision for a dramatic career change. He wrote later that "if I were to devote myself to the improvement of a degraded profession, closely connected with the interest of agriculture, I might render myself much more useful to the country, than by continuing in one already cultivated by men of the most splendid talents."[xix] By "a degraded profession" he meant veterinary medicine.

John Lyon tried hard to persuade Moorcroft to leave off his mad scheme of trading a surgeon's profession to be a lowly veterinarian and even sent him off to talk to **John Hunter** in 1788, who was the leading surgeon in London in his day. But Hunter ended up supporting the young Moorcroft, saying, "If I were not so advanced in years, I myself would begin on the following day to study the profession in question."[xx]

John Hunter (1728-1793) was a brilliant English surgeon who performed influential experimentation and writing in the field of comparative anatomy and physiology. Among his extensive research were important studies on wound healing and inflammation in dogs. He was born a poor farmer's son and orphaned as a child. At 20 years old he lived and trained with his brother William, who eventually became England's best surgeon. He was a military surgeon for the British army during the Seven Years' War. He encouraged William Jenner to produce the smallpox vaccine from cowpox (the hide of Bessie, the cow that originated the cowpox vaccine, hung in his amazing private medical museum). Hunter argued for the establishment of a veterinary school in England and encouraged William Moorcroft to go to veterinary school.

John Hunter went on the next year to lobby for the creation of an English vet school. It was founded in London in 1791 with the help of the Odiham Agriculture Society of Hampshire and dubbed simply "The Veterinary College, London." Significantly, it was the voice of a clergyman-farmer named Thomas Burgess, pointing out the inhumane and unscientific practices of farriers in his day and the need for better agricultural practices, which first sparked the Odiham Society's interest in a veterinary school.[xxi] We see again the recurring theme of Christian clergymen taking an active interest in the welfare and medicine of animals. The Earl of Pembroke became involved in the school, as part of his campaign to improve the quality of life among army horses. John Hunter and Royal Society president Sir Joseph Banks were among the first members of the board. The school became the Royal College of Veterinary Medicine after it received a Royal charter in 1875.

But when the London school was founded, Moorcroft was away. He went to Lyon to study in the momentous year of 1789 when France was broiling with revolutionary feelings ready to erupt into the Reign of Terror. The school was declining by then. The four-year program, compressed to a single year of study, had only two faculty members listed (Louis Bedin and Jacques-Marie Henon). Moorcroft spent the year studying anatomy, animal husbandry, medicine, and pathology.

When he returned home in 1792, William started a practice in equine medicine, which flourished wildly. Society in his day depended on horses for many things, from agriculture to sports to transportation. Moorcroft's excellent educational and agricultural background made him uniquely suited to run the first solidly scientific-based veterinary practice in England. He started an equine hospital on Oxford Street in London and practiced successfully. He also taught at the new veterinary college. However, William "became disgusted with his occupation, although he speedily realized a handsome property by it."[xxii] Moorcroft's career was about to undergo another dramatic change!

Amid a flurry of patriotism birthed out of the fear of Napoleon invading England, Moorcroft joined a company of volunteers (the Westminster Volunteer Cavalry) in 1803. His work in the cavalry impressed Edward Parry of the East India Company, who talked Moorcroft into becoming manager of the stud (breeding) program for the Company's India office. The East India Company had grown from a small group of traders to a massive international operation, big enough to conduct its own wars. An operation that big needed a lot of horsepower. And in India in particular, the company needed bigger, stronger horses to carry soldiers and equipment over rough terrain—stronger horses than they could find in India. So they sent Moorcroft to produce better horses with their breeding program. In 1808 Moorcroft took the perilous journey to British Calcutta and improved the East India Company's stud program dramatically over the next few years. By 1811 he started traveling far distances to cities such as Lucknow to search for better stock.

In 1812 Moorcroft and a friend named Captain William Hearsey disguised themselves as Hindu pilgrims, then bartered their way into Tibet. The remarkable expedition comprehensively explored uncharted territory few westerners had seen. They were even granted authority to trade in cashmere (expensive wool from a special breed of goat), and to explore Lake Manasarovar, high in the Tibetan mountains, fed by glaciers, and still held as sacred by several religions in the region. None of this impressed the East India Company, who were angry at Moorcroft for failing to find horses to breed. They denied Moorcroft's request for funding to explore Bukhara (modern-day Uzbekistan, Tajikistan, Turkmenistan, and Kazakhstan).

Moorcroft sent Persian-born Mir Izzat-Allah to map Bukhara after being told about the fine horses there. He particularly wanted to get a rumored breed of horse called the Turkoman horses (Akhal-Teke by locals), which Marco Polo had written about in the 13th century. It was said Turkomans were exceptionally hardy and beautiful. After seven years of nagging the East India Company, Moorcroft got permission to look for them. He took nearly a year to put together an extensive and expensive caravan (comprising about 300 members along with 12 Gurkha guides) and set off in 1820. The caravan made it as far as the Buddhist kingdom of Ladakh where they were delayed for nearly two years awaiting permission to journey onward (both by the local government and by the Company, who were unhappy about Moorcroft overstepping his authority to propose a trade treaty with a Sikh Maharaja). Moorcroft used this time to explore the area of Ladakh, a part of Kashmir lying west of Tibet. William pressed on in lobbying

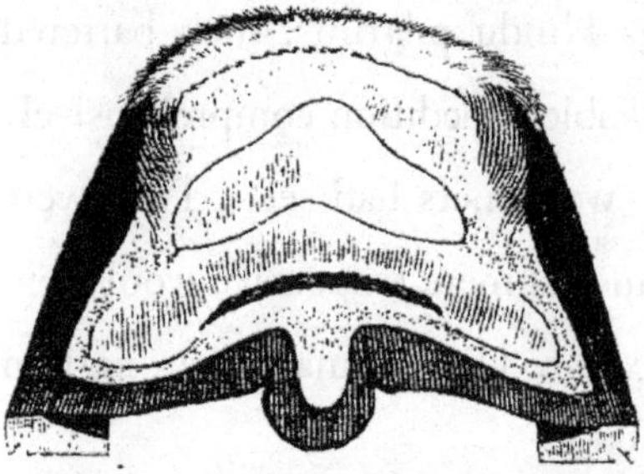

Diagram of a horse hoof in cross-section from a book William Moorcroft wrote and published, in an effort to improve horse-shoeing practices of his day.

for further exploration with dogged determination, writing in one letter, "I must push the adventure to the end."[xxiii] The expedition eventually made its way as far as Kabul, exploring many wonders previously unseen by European eyes. During his travels, he also used his surgical training to offer clinics for locals afflicted with conditions like cataracts and wounds and goiter.

Though historians are still uncertain, William Moorcroft probably did more than explore Tibet and India. England and Russia in his day were at diplomatic odds with each other over relations with Afghanistan and the surrounding regions. A shadowy confrontation between the two nations, often called "the Great Game," pitted Russian and English explorers fighting for trade rights and better relations with central Asian peoples. There is evidence the patriotic Moorcroft spied for England on the activity of Russian explorers, providing intelligence about Russia's relations with Tibet.[xxiv] His intelligence gathering was not without risk. The East India Company declared and led war against the Gorkha kings, who invaded Nepal and prompted a confederation of native states to ask the Company for help. The Anglo-Nepalese War lasted from 1814 to 1816, and Moorcroft gathered intelligence for the movement of troops as well as trade.

Though he traveled far, Moorcroft never found the Turkoman horses. Sadly, he died of fever in 1825 in Turkestan—at least we think so. Some believed he faked his death and retired.

William Moorcroft wrote meticulously about his travels but was not very verbose about his faith in the writings he left behind (at least those I've read). But he was certainly the product of a nation tinted with Christian beliefs and wrote from a standpoint of Christian faith. In one part of his descriptions of Kashmir, he recommended bringing the Christian gospel to a people he described as being oppressed into poverty by Hindu and Muslim governments. "There seems, indeed, to be little attachment of either the Mohammedans or Hindus of Kashmir to their respective creeds, and I am convinced there is no part of India where the pure religion of the Gospel might be introduced with a fairer prospect of success."[xxv]

One reads no hints of sarcasm in Moorcroft's use of the phrase "the pure religion of the Gospel," and this certainly sounds like the words of a man who loved Christ!

Meanwhile, in England, others were continuing veterinary research and teaching at the Royal Veterinary College. **Delabere Blaine** (1770-1845) was one of the first appointed professors at the college. He trained as a surgeon for seven years before he attended medical school and worked under Dr. Haighton, who was researching neurophysiology using dogs as a model. He drew important anatomical sketches of Haighton's method of nerve transection for pain relief in the dog.

Because of Blaine's work, Sainbel (an emigrant from France who helped found the new veterinary college) appointed him to teach anatomy, physiology, and pathology. Sadly, the irascible Sainbel fired him not long after. Blaine practiced veterinary medicine on his own and became influential in canine medicine, which was neglected in his age in favor of the more useful horse. He did work for a time as an equine surgeon for the Royal Horse Artillery. He never officially earned a veterinary degree but practiced successfully, something which brought disdain from contemporary veterinarians. He published several influential books on canine medicine and became an important founder in companion animal medicine, including a monumental work on canine distemper published in 1800 and a general *Canine Pathology* published in 1817. He declined an offer as director of the veterinary school in St. Petersburg, Russia.

Blaine took veterinarian **William Youatt** (1776-1847) first as an apprentice around 1813, and eventually as a partner, and their practice grew to see about 2-3k canine cases per year, along with some equine cases.

Youatt did not become a veterinarian until the age of 37. He was the son of a nonconformist minister (one not adhering to the Church of England) and trained as a minister early in life. He worked as a pastor in London, where he developed an interest in animal medicine. At Blaine's insistence, William attended the London Veterinary College for veterinary qualifications, but was driven out by Principal Coleman, who disliked him

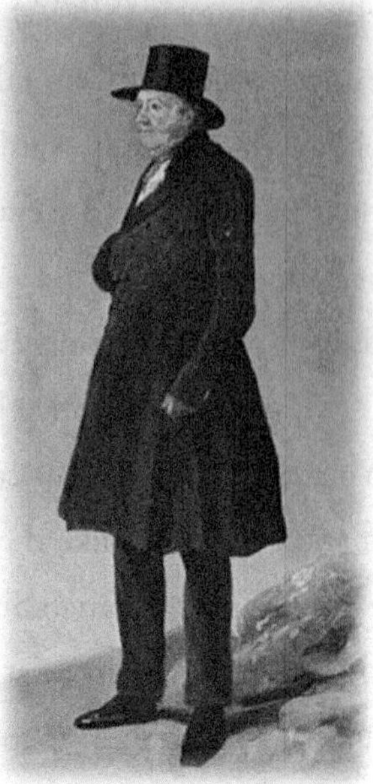

Portrait of William Youatt, by Richard Ansdell

for his association with Blaine. After Coleman died, Youatt officially completed his degree in veterinary medicine in 1844.

In 1839 he published a book on animal welfare called *The Obligation and Extent of Humanity to Brutes*, which rekindled the old debate about whether animals have souls. In it, he referred to man as a created being, appealed to Scripture and the moral law of nature, making multiple references in his writing to Jesus as "our Savior." The entire first section ("The Obligation of Humanity to Animals as Founded on the Scriptures") is an eloquent argument from the Bible that people should take good care of animals and not be cruel to them.

This Christian interest in animal welfare is further illustrated by Youatt's participation in the Society for the Prevention of Cruelty to Animals (SPCA) essay contest which specifically required essays "which shall morally illustrate, and religiously enforce, the obligation of man towards the inferior and dependent creatures—their protection and security from abuse… Humanity to the brute as harmonious with the spirit and doctrines of Christianity, and the duty of man as a rational and accountable creature."[xxvi]

There was an active interest among Christians in England in Youatt's day to prevent cruelty to animals, which sparked the formation of groups like the SPCA—who appointed Youatt as their Honorary Veterinarian Surgeon in 1835. Youatt illustrated the fact that much of this interest was based on a Biblical understanding of animal welfare in his book introduction, where he quoted the Society for the Suppression of Cruelty. "He who professes to honour his Maker no longer dares openly to sanction cruelty to the brute creation... The pure sincere advocacy of the animal world is passionless and disinterested; working out that beautiful principle of Christian charity, which, having been given to a man in perfect love, is thus to be extended to the meanest of God's creatures."[xxvii]

These principles, almost straight from the words of Proverbs 12:10, helped meld William Youatt, the nonconformist minister, into William Youatt, the veterinarian. And there is little doubt they were the same principles that motivated him often in his clinical practice and research.

William was a busy writer. He edited the first veterinary professional journal, *The Veterinarian.* He also published a series of books on the medicine of all the popular domestic animals in his day. Youatt was an early proponent of broadening veterinary medicine to include all species and worked to improve the public respectability of the profession. Ironically, both Youatt and Blaine were far ahead of the more respectable and "ivory tower" Coleman in their ideas of disease and contagion. They did important research on rabies in particular. Youatt also had a strong agricultural influence and was involved in livestock medicine.

Tragically William Youatt committed suicide in 1847, after years of battling chronic depression. Despite this sad end Youatt stands tall (along with his colleague Delabare Blaine) as an exceptionally compassionate veterinarian, informed and inspired by Christian principles, and among the first to truly broaden the profession's focus toward care for all animal species.

"The Creator loves the animals he made, called them good, and made humanity his emissaries on earth to care for them. Where these Christian teachings have been taken seriously throughout history, we see Christians make real efforts to alleviate animal suffering and cure animal disease."

Veterinarians Today

There is so much more we could explore in the long story of veterinary medicine's development. There is the transplantation of professional veterinary medicine to North America (through the influence of Scottish and British veterinarians into Canada, spreading from there into the United States). There is the development of the profession through revolutionary scientific discoveries during the 20th century. And of course, the influence of the Christian faith is present in all these eras. That influence continues in the profession currently, alive and busy with the work of God's kingdom through the care of animals.

Today, an extensive and international group of veterinarians works around the world, not only to care for animals but to spread Christ's gospel by doing it. A Georgian veterinarian named Dr. Leroy Dorminy started **Christian Veterinary Mission** in 1976. A woman from an underdeveloped part of Africa inspired him to start the organization. As he spoke to her at a Baptist conference in Stockholm, Sweden, he asked what he could do for her homeland. She told him it needed somebody to teach veterinary skills so people could take care of their animals. Later turned away by a mission group, he realized there was no specific outlet in mission work for utilizing his skill set as a veterinarian. And so he started an organization to do just that.

The group describes its purpose succinctly on the main page of its website. "Christian Veterinary Mission exists to share the love of Christ through veterinary medicine. Working in communities worldwide, CVM equips and encourages veterinary professionals and students to build relationships with others through the use of their veterinary knowledge and skills so that lives are transformed."[xxviii] What a wonderful goal for every Christian veterinarian, whether or not they go overseas on the mission field!

But the primary purpose of this history section is to examine Christianity's influence on the birth of the profession in particular. We've seen how the ideas of Scripture have inspired many scientists and clinicians (both professional and amateur) who were influential in the birth of veterinary medicine as a specific discipline. Sometimes the Bible directly influenced their reflections and motivations, and sometimes the Christian culture in which they lived more indirectly influenced them.

None of this should come as a surprise. The Creator loves the animals he made, called them good, and made humanity his emissaries on earth to care for them. Where these Christian teachings have been taken seriously throughout history, we see Christians make genuine efforts to ease animal suffering and cure animal disease.

– II –

Christian Theology of Veterinary Medicine

Why were so many Christians involved in the formative years of veterinary medicine? How would their faith have inspired them to dedicate so much time and effort to animal wellbeing? Does the Bible have something to say about animal medicine?

Yes! The Bible does address the topic of veterinary medicine. The exact words "veterinary medicine" aren't found in the Bible. But a careful reading of Scripture will direct your thinking about A) the status of animal life in relation to human life and B) our moral obligations as humans toward animals.

In this section, we will look at how Christians ought to think about animals and animal wellbeing.

God Cares for Animals

> *"God must respect life and care about animals... He cannot be cruel."*

An important starting place in any examination of theology is the mind of God. The word theology, after all, literally means "the study of God." What does the Creator think about the animals He made?

The answer is simple to find: the Bible shows God cares about animal wellbeing. Indeed, as pastor and veterinarian William Youatt wrote of the Bible: "There is no other book in the world, which, not written expressly on the duties of humanity, breathes so affectionate a spirit towards these dumb members of God's great family below [animals], and gives so remarkable a prominence to subjects connected with their welfare."[xxix]

Scripture addresses God's care for animals from its first pages. When God made the world, he called the fish and birds and land animals very good. Here's an important logical argument we can conclude about God's nature from Genesis: God is good; respect for life is a quality of goodness; animals are living things. And thus, God must respect life and care about animals. Granted, the reason we know "a respect of all of life is a quality of goodness" is precisely because God, who is the ultimate definition of all that's good, declared life to be "very good" in Genesis. C. S. Lewis wrote a very similar argument in *The Problem of Pain*: "From the doctrine that God is good we may confidently deduce that the *appearance* of reckless Divine cruelty in the animal kingdom is an illusion."[xxx]

God cannot be cruel. He is gentle, and he treats *all living things* with a special gentility.

After creating the animals, God brought them (not the rocks and plants) to Adam to be named because they were special, in a category above non-living things. He put man in charge to "subdue" and "have dominion" over animals (Genesis 1:28), but he did not give us animals as food or as slaves. It is significant that God originally gave "every plant yielding seed" and tree to mankind for food, and also gave the same plants and trees to animal-kind, "that has the breath of life" (Genesis 1:29-30). He elevates all living things, man and animals, to a status above any non-living thing. He pronounces the blood that pumps through living things to be unique in creation, and not to be eaten by his people in the Old Testament (Leviticus 17:11).

David declared in Psalm 36:6 that God saves man "and beast." He preserves animal-kind and takes care of them. In Psalm 145:9 he declares God's compassion extends to "all that he has made." Notice this is written in the context of praise to God. The fact of God's concern about the animal kingdom should generate more than mere intellectual discussion: it should be another reason to admire our wonderful heavenly Father, who cares for every one of His creatures. Praise the gentle God, who loves life and cares for it everywhere!

"Praise the gentle God, who loves life and cares for it everywhere!"

Jesus told us He is the image of His father, and when we see Him, we see God. In Jesus, we see vast amounts of gentle kindness—toward people, certainly, but also toward animals. In an ancient world culture that considered animals exclusively as objects (to be worked, or eaten, or slaughtered on an altar, or fought in arenas for entertainment) this really is remarkable. In Matthew 10:29, Christ famously declared that not a single sparrow falls to the ground "apart from your Father." We tend to read this passage only for the conclusion that God cares more for us than the sparrows (which is indeed correct). But we can't forget the clear implication that God cares for the sparrows. When arguing with the Pharisees about exceptions to keeping the Sabbath day rest, Christ chose to make an exception for injured animals (pointing out even the Pharisees would pull their injured sheep from a ditch on the Sabbath). The context of this passage should be considered. In the next verse, Christ asks *"of how much more value is a man than a sheep?"* (Matthew 12:11-12). We'll talk about the value of human life over animal life a bit later. But for now, notice the gentility of a Savior who preaches God's concern for animal life in a Roman world famous for harsh violence.

In Jonah 4:11, God parenthetically tells Jonah that he should care about the 120,000 people in Nineveh *and also the animals.* God gives thought to all life in Nineveh, not only the human life, and implies it would be tragic for the animals to die.

"...a characteristic of a righteous man is caring for animals. A characteristic of a wicked man is cruelty to animals."

In Numbers 22:28 we read about God's use of an unusual messenger. Balaam's donkey saw an angel when Balaam could not, and "the Lord opened the mouth of the donkey" and she complained and spoke to her master. The words not chosen in this verse are fascinating. Scripture does not say "the Lord put words into the donkey's mouth" or "the Lord spoke through the donkey." It simply says He opened her mouth. This would imply that the donkey had thoughts before God opened her mouth to express them to Balaam! She understood the situation, knew Balaam was about to walk to his death, and needed a warning. God merely opened her mouth so that she could communicate those thoughts to her master.

There is a mystery here. We see clues that Balaam's donkey is a thinking being, but we are not told any more than that by Scripture. However, the mere possibility that animals may have a more complex consciousness than we know ought to make a world of difference in the way we treat them. If a beast might have a sort of corporeal soul, a center of thought and feeling more complex or "higher" than we realize, then we might well be morally culpable for cruelty to him. But whether Balaam's donkey was expressing anything like cogent self-realization, it is plain the angel rebuked Balaam for beating the donkey (Numbers 22:32). God does not like cruelty to animals. Much to the contrary, his gentle voice makes the deer give birth (Psalm 29:9). He cares about all life.

"The great Maker of all has delegated to man a portion of his authority," wrote William Youatt, "but he has not withdrawn his

---

"The mere possibility that animals may have a more complex consciousness than we know, ought to make a world of difference in the way we treat them."

---

watchful care from one of his creatures. How often and how beautifully is this illustrated in the sacred volume!"[xxxi]

We Should Care for Animals

If God cares about the well-being of animals, one would expect Him to teach his people to care for animals as well. And that is precisely what we find in Scripture.

We find the plainest instance of God commanding kindness to animals in Proverbs 12:10, a verse I've been pleased to find printed on boxes from veterinary drug companies before. *"Whoever is righteous has regard for the life of his beast, but the mercy of the wicked is cruel."*

Solomon, under the inspiration of the Holy Spirit, tells us that a characteristic of a righteous man is caring for animals. A characteristic of a wicked man is cruelty to animals. Human beings are not free to treat animals any way they want. Rather, humans have a moral responsibility to treat the animals under our care with gentility. On Judgement Day, God will ask you about how well you cared for the animals you interacted with.

Matthew Henry commented, "He regards even *the life of his beast,* not only because it is his servant, but because it is God's creature, and in conformity to Providence, which *preserves man and beast.* The beasts that are under our care must be provided for, must have convenient food and rest, must in no case be abused or tyrannised over."

Chuck Smith echoed these same thoughts in more simple terms: "Kindness to animals is a sign of a righteous man. A person who is cruel to an animal is really cruel to one of God's creatures, one of God's creation. So the righteous man regards the life of his beast."[xxxii]

The Hebrew word for "the life" means a breathing creature, with blood in its veins, and carries echoes of God's sanctifying words about lifeblood in the law of Leviticus 17:11 ("the life of the flesh is in the blood"). It also carries a connotation of the self or even the soul, the center of emotions and passions. It is perfectly consistent with Scripture, and with historic Christian teaching, to affirm animals have thoughts and feelings.

The Hebrew for "regards" in Proverbs 12:10 particularly implies knowledge, and this is a large part of the domain of veterinary medicine. The work of a veterinarian is the application of knowledge to the promotion of animal health. The optimal ability to fight animal disease and promote animal wellbeing requires detailed knowledge in a wide range of subjects. Animal anatomy, physiology, animal husbandry, pathophysiology, nutrition, pharmacodynamics are only a few of these. One of the major applications of Proverbs 12:10 for veterinarians is that it takes work to understand our patients and the diseases they face, in order to show genuine regard for their well-being.

Solomon, the divinely inspired author of most of the Proverbs, had a special interest in nature, and in animals in particular. *"He spoke also of beasts, and of birds, and of reptiles, and of fish"* (1 Kings 4:33b). So perhaps it's not very surprising to find that the passages dealing most directly with animal welfare in Scripture were by Solomon.

In Proverbs 27:23 that wise king wrote, *"Know well the condition of your flocks, and give attention to your herds."* Although a major point of this passage is a lesson in diligence and economic wisdom in an agriculturally based society, it also admonishes care for the health of the animals under one's supervision. Agricultural endeavors (often termed "animal husbandry") have been a means of motivating people to care for animals from the earliest times to the present. Here Solomon observes that if you take good care of your sheep, they will take good care of you (v. 26). Here also is a motivation for the scientific, medical theory behind veterinary medicine. We are to *know* the state of our flocks. Good care requires accurate knowledge.

Many of the Old Testament laws, given by God particularly for Israel, reflect his concern for animal wellbeing. God includes domestic animals in the Sabbath rest proscribed for His people (Exodus 20:10). He commands Israelites to return stray animals (Exodus 23:4) and to help over-burdened animals wherever they are found, even in the herds of enemies (Exodus 23:5). God tells Israelites not to take birds away from brooding their eggs (Deuteronomy 22:6). He commands against the cruelty of boiling a goat kid in its mother's milk (Exodus 23:19). He tells Israelites to even the load of animals pulling plows (Deuteronomy 25:4), which would help protect them from pressure sores and some chronic musculoskeletal conditions, as well as making their job easier. These commands to God's Old Testament people are all practical methods of exercising care toward animal life, amid the backdrop of ancient world cultures which often tended toward cruelty. They are also expressions of His gentility toward animals.

Animal Sacrifices

What about animal sacrifices God commanded His people in the Old Testament to perform? Does the cruel act of slaughtering animals on an altar negate the passages of the Bible which talk about being kind to animals? This is a tough question. But the answer lies in a proper understanding of the nature and context of the sacrifices proscribed by the Old Testament Levitical law.

Animal sacrifice was for the atonement of sin but acknowledged to be a terrible act. That was largely the point. The fall, the brokenness of a perfect creation, made a terrible act of substitutionary death needful that shouldn't have been necessary. God showed Israel the terrible consequences of their sins through animal sacrifice. We humans tend to take sin lightly, especially when we're the ones doing it. From the very beginning of Scripture we read sin brings death (Genesis

"Creation should thrive under our watchful and diligent hands."

3:3, 19). Sin doesn't just make God angry. It has death-dealing consequences and brings sorrow and misery to society by its very nature. And part of the horror of sin was supposed to be shown in the Old Testament horror of sacrificing animals.

These sacrifices were part of the spiritual reality that sin demands atonement. More specifically, that sin demands blood atonement (Romans 6:23). This is communicated in Leviticus 17:11 as the point of animal sacrifice in the Old Testament Law. *"For the life of the flesh is in the blood, and I have given it for you on the altar to make atonement for your souls, for it is the blood that makes atonement by the life."*

That's why the writers of the New Testament often write about how animal sacrifices under the old Levitical law were a picture of the ultimate and comprehensive sacrifice of Christ on the cross. When Jesus, the perfect God-man died for sin, the Israelites could stop the terrible and ongoing practice of animal sacrifices at last. Jesus' sacrifice was perfect and comprehensive and did away with the need for any further sacrifice at all. We can be thankful for that!

The purpose of animal sacrifice in Old Testament Israel, it should be noted, differed greatly from the purpose of animal sacrifices in other ancient cultures surrounding Israel. Most cultures in the ancient world (like the Greeks, the Egyptians, the Mesopotamians, and the Aztecs) practiced animal sacrifices. But they meant their sacrifices to appease an angry god, prevent some kind of natural disaster, or tell the future. Israel's sacrifices, while atoning for sin, were especially meant to be a picture: a picture of the terrible consequence of sin, and a picture of better things to come under Christ. Israel's sacrifices are presented in Scripture as a "necessary evil," something that God might be imagined weeping over—and something He expected His people to weep over. Their presence in Scripture does not mean that God is not gentle and does not care about animal life.

Dominion

We should look at the admonition to care for animals under our supervision in light of the theological concept of *dominion.* The "dominion mandate" is the Biblical teaching that God put mankind in charge of the rest of creation. Even the Hebrew word translated "give attention to" in Proverbs 27:23 carries a connotation of ruling.

This was part of the original order of creation found in Genesis. *"Then God said, 'Let us make man in our image, after our likeness. And let them have dominion over the fish of the sea and over the birds of the heavens and over the livestock and over all the earth and over every creeping thing that creeps on the earth'"* (Gen. 1:26).

God made mankind to rule creation. This is a creation reality expressed in the Bible, not just a social construct. The words are repeated several times in Genesis and other passages as well (such as Psalm 8:6-8). Dr. Henry Morris writes of the creation order, "This was God's first commandment to the man and woman He had created. They were to exercise dominion 'over all the earth' (v. 26); not a despotic dominion, as some have insinuated, but a responsible stewardship."[xxxiii] God made us to be kings and queens over creation.

In this ruling we are not to be tyrants. In Genesis 2:15 we see the dominion call of man in the command to "work" and to "keep" the Garden of Eden. The Hebrew word for "to keep" carries the connotation of catching and guarding and preserving, as well as ruling. The major thrust of the dominion mandate is that people are meant to *care for* nature. God made us to tend it. His plan is that creation should thrive under our watchful and diligent hands. As I wrote in another book, "We are to tend the garden: to take this earth we live on and make it better by our hard work and rule. We are to follow God's lead and stamp our creative handiwork on his creation, making it more beautiful than it was before. This is an exciting calling!"[xxxiv]

"Caring for sick animals is part of reversing the sad effects of the fall. It's part of the great battle against death and suffering that Christ calls us to as redeemed people."

Ruling brings responsibility. C. S. Lewis wrote in his essay on animal suffering, "Man was appointed by God to have dominion over the beasts, and everything a man does to an animal is either a lawful exercise, or a sacrilegious abuse, of an authority by Divine right."[xxxv]

The Bible expands the concept of dominion in the soteriology (study of salvation) of the Old and New Testaments. It teaches that all creation fell with the fall of man, its ruler. Adam and Eve's first sin ushered in the curse of death and suffering and misery, which was not part of the original plan for life on earth. It's vital we understand that death and suffering (in all living things) are foreign to God's original creation. They are evil, injected from the outside, by the Prince of Evil, into perfect order. The animal kingdom was never intended to be "red in tooth and claw" as Tennyson once described it. But Christ's work of salvation reversed the effects of the fall, and not just in a spiritual sense.

"For the creation waits with eager longing for the revealing of the sons of God. For the creation was subjected to futility, not willingly, but because of him who subjected it, in hope that the creation itself will be set free from its bondage to corruption and obtain the freedom of the glory of the children of God" (Romans 8:19-21).

Jesus crushed the power of Satan and started the great march toward a new creation. He began the work of reversing the side-effects of sin—death, misery, and suffering—which will one day be gone entirely. His redeemed people are his hands and feet in that work. He uses our efforts to wage war on the unnatural suffering and death that plagues this sin-ravaged world. This has been an important Christian motive for scientific research and medicine in the past and is a good motive for practicing veterinary medicine in particular. Caring for sick animals is an important part of reversing the sad effects of the fall.

We, as human beings, are created to rule creation in the image of our loving and gentle God. We are called to treat animals with gentility. And even more, we're called to actively fight against what harms them. A high part of our calling as kings of creation is to care for life, work to alleviate suffering, and promote animal health and well-being. This applies in a special way to redeemed human beings, who should be conscious about their participation in the great work of their Savior in reversing the effects of Adam's fall.

The unfallen world was a world without animal suffering. And, though it may never be something we'll see again this side of paradise, we can work toward that goal in real ways as veterinarians, and as responsible pet owners.

An idea we often don't consider is that pet ownership itself is not a result of the fall. There are many ways sin distorted the human-animal relationship, just like it distorted animal and human health by introducing disease. C.S. Lewis contrasts the idea of the tame animal being in its natural state to the atheistic idea that a wild animal is the most natural of animals. "The tame animal is therefore, in the deepest sense, the only 'natural' animal—the only one we see occupying the place it was made to occupy, and it is on the tame animal that we must base all our doctrine of beasts."[xxxvi] If, by "natural," we mean "closest to the first ordering of things in the original creation," then a Bible-based view of animal-kind should agree with Lewis. The most natural animal is one under the control of benevolent human rule. Wild animals (who sometimes even attack humans), or humans who abuse animals, are visible effects of the perversion of what is natural. A vision for a perfect world should include a harmonious relationship of humans with animals, as well as a world in which suffering and disease are minimized.

Is Fifi Immortal?

Do animals have souls? Will my dog, or cat, or crawdad, or lizard go to heaven when they die? It's a much more complicated theological question than many Christians imagine and is one the Bible does not speak directly on.

The prevailing, orthodox position of the historic Church has always been that animals are fundamentally different than humans, and do not go to heaven.

Much of the Scriptural argument for this idea rests in the observation from Genesis that God created man in the image of God (Genesis 1:26). Intellect and will in particular are part of the image of God that mankind was built specially to reflect. John Piper, writing about Habakkuk 2:14, points out that man fills the unique role in creation of praising God in a knowledgeable, intellectual way. "In one sense, nature itself fills the earth with the glory of the Lord. But that is not the ultimate goal. For God's purpose in creation to be attained, there must be a world filled with the '*knowledge* of the glory of the Lord.' Trees may clap their hands for God (Isa. 55:12), but they do not know what they are doing. Such conscious, joyful knowing, loving, and praising is the destiny of man, not nature. The goal of creation is not simply the echo of God's excellence in the exulting fields (Ps. 96:12), the rejoicing crocuses (Isa. 35:1), the singing mountains (Isa. 55:12), and the hand-clapping rivers (Ps. 98:8). The goal is the echo of God's excellence in the perceiving minds and praising hearts of human beings created in his image."[xxxvii]

But it is important to understand that "God's image" is a comprehensive, ethereal, and theological description of what makes human beings special—one which encompasses more than just the sense of reason or the ability to choose right and wrong. God's image in us is more than intellect and will.

John Calvin pointed out in his commentary on Genesis: "Thus the chief seat of the Divine image was in his mind and heart, where it was eminent: yet was there no part of him in which some scintillations of it did not shine forth."[xxxviii] In other words, God's image is part of the whole man. It is something we believe we have because Scripture tells us we have it, even though it's difficult to pinpoint and describe. The divine image is spoken of as an almost mysterious substance that permeates every part of a human being (not just his reasoning mind) *and sets him apart from animal-kind.* This is important to the present discussion because animals do show thoughts and emotions, heads and hearts. But it does not follow that they carry the "image of God." If the divine image is, as the church has taught over the centuries, a part of the whole man, the words of Genesis 1:26 make more sense. And, in the historic teaching of the church, it is the divine image inside of us that will live forever. This is usually what we mean by man's soul in theology.

John Gill echoed the orthodox teachings of the church when he wrote that the image of God in man *is the basis for the immortality of the soul.* "The soul of man is made after the image, and in the likeness of God, which chiefly consists in that; it bears a resemblance to the divine nature being the breath of God; it has a likeness to him, and particularly in its immortality."[xxxix]

That last phrase is important to the present discussion. It's the image of God, the soul, which lives forever and cannot die. The corporeal part of a being (the body, the flesh) will die. But the incorporeal soul will not. Because animals don't share in the image of God, they are only corporeal bodies. Though Scripture does not speak directly on the subject, Christianity from its inception has reasoned from passages like Genesis 1:26 that animals do not have souls (as God did not make them in His image), and are only corporeal. This would mean individual animals do not go to heaven when they die. When they die, they are gone.

Early Dissenters

Since the Bible does not *directly* tell us if animals will go to Heaven, there have been orthodox (non-heretical) Christian thinkers as early as the 4th century AD who thought animals would resurrect and go to heaven. One can be a Bible-believing Christian and safely believe that animals will be in heaven.

We find anecdotal evidence of Christian belief in animal resurrection in art and archeology. For example, among a depiction of the resurrection in the mosaics at the cathedral at Torcello (by Venice) one can see resurrected animals.[xl] We also see this in the writings of some major Christian thinkers.

There were several ways in which some founders of church doctrine included animals in the ranks of those blessed in heaven. The Biblical idea that flesh will rise (as well as our souls) in the last days was an important theological foundation for this position. One idea, propounded by some early church fathers (such as St. Irenaeus and a minority of medieval thinkers) included resurrected animals among all of creation which would resurrect on the last day. They argued that because the flesh will rise on the last day, animals (being corporeal) might be included.

Another view bases the idea of animals going to heaven on the general renewing of all creation. Historian Joyce Salisbury wrote about this historic Christian view of animal resurrection. "Some people saw God's creation as a unity, a great web in which all are linked together in this world, and transformed into the next. In this view, the question is not whether animals would go to heaven, but whether a whole environmental web of creation might be risen to an afterlife."[xli]

This echoes Paul's teaching in Romans 8:22-23 that "all

creation" is waiting for the resurrection. *"For we know that the whole creation has been groaning together in the pains of childbirth until now. And not only creation, but we ourselves, who have the firstfruits of the Spirit, groan inwardly as we wait eagerly for adoption as sons, the redemption of our bodies."*[xlii]

Animal-kind certainly is part of the whole creation. What is more, as we've seen already, animal-kind is more important than some parts of all creation (more valuable than non-life). Surely, if God intends to raise all creation, he will include all living parts. Paul also mentions here that we as humans have "the firstfruits of the Spirit." This might be taken as evidence for C. S. Lewis's intriguing theory of animal resurrection based on their interaction with redeemed humans.

The C. S. Lewis Hypothesis

Lewis propounded a unique idea about animal souls and immortality in his book *The Problem of Pain.* He starts his discussion by adding to the medieval debate about animal sentience (ability to think), clarifying an important distinction between sentience and consciousness, to reinforce the idea that animals do not have souls. "But at this level we must still distinguish sentience from consciousness… Suppose that three sensations follow one another first A, then B, then C. When this happens to you, you have the experience of passing through the process ABC. But note what this implies. It implies there is something in you which stands sufficiently outside

A to notice A passing away, and sufficiently outside B to notice B now beginning and coming to fill the place which A has vacated; and something which recognises itself as the same through the transition from A to B and B to C so that it can say 'I have had the experience ABC.' ... Now it is almost certain that the nervous system of one of the higher animals presents it with successive sensations. It does not follow that it has any 'soul', anything which recognises itself as having had A, and now having B, and now marking how B glides away to make room for C. If it had no such 'soul,' what we call the experience ABC would never occur."[xliii]

A bit later in the essay Lewis (taking the side of most Christian philosophers) clarifies that this lack of consciousness in most animals bears directly on their immortality. "The real difficulty about supposing most animals to be immortal is that immortality has almost no meaning for a creature which is not 'conscious' in the sense explained above... There is, therefore, I take it, no question of immortality for creatures that are merely sentient.'[xliv]

So far this is just a reasoned expression of the historic church teaching that animals lack a soul, and will therefore not resurrect. But Lewis adds an interesting theory, rooted in the dominion mandate expressed in Genesis. He admits that there may be a gradient of animal consciousness: there are "higher animals" who seem to have some sense of self, or that we at least attribute personality to. Then he discusses how this personality invariably comes from the animal's interaction with a human while being tamed. An animal might gain selfhood, personality, sentience in relation to the human it lives with. And, according to the prevailing views of the historic church, this could imply immortality. "Man is to be understood only in his relation to God. The beasts are to be understood only in their relation to man and, through man, to God."[xlv]

In a similar, mysterious way that redeemed humans are "in Christ" (that is, represented by Christ, and partakers of His identity), Lewis hypothesizes our family pet might be said to be "in us." Being in Christ assures our place in heaven. What if being in us ensures our pet's place? "And in this way it seems to me possible that certain animals may have an immortality, not in themselves, but in the immortality of their masters."[xlvi] Lewis would say animals lack souls, but that some animals can attain immortality by imputation from redeemed humans. This is a theory argued from broad ideas in Scripture, and not at all directly taught by Scripture. It is very speculative as Lewis himself declares, since it is about a topic we can only make informed guesses about.

But his imputation theory of animal immortality has merit. It "makes God the centre of the universe and man the subordinate centre of terrestrial nature: the beasts are not co-ordinate with man, but subordinate to him, and their destiny is through and through related to his."[xlvii]

– III –

Christian Philosophy of Veterinary Medicine

God is not silent on the importance of animal wellbeing—which is the primary interest of the veterinary practitioner. But Scripture does not speak on some topics related to animal health. Can we use reason, working inductively from what the Bible says and from what we can observe in nature, to answer these important questions?

In this section, we'll look at what Christian philosophers have said about important topics like the nature of animals, the possibility of a soul in animal-kind, and the ethics of prohibiting animal cruelty. Philosophy can scare some readers. But remember that philosophy is "the handmaiden of theology," as Thomas Aquinas wrote (quoting Clement of Alexandria). It is a practical tool for thinking deeply about the concepts of Scripture considering the actual world we live in.

The ideas of the 13th century Christian philosopher Thomas Aquinas have perhaps been the most influential among philosophic writers in shaping the historic Christian view of animals. Aquinas' ideas about animal life are rooted in the writings of older philosophers (like Augustine and Aristotle) as well as in Scripture. We will discuss their ideas primarily in this section.

Thomist philosophers (ones who agree with Aquinas) divide living things into three groups to describe a kind of hierarchy of life. There is vegetative life on one level (the plants), then more complex animal life a step up, then rational life (human life) as an even more complex step up. All vegetable life has several abilities: the ability to eat (to take in the non-living matter and incorporate it into living matter), to grow, and to reproduce. Animal life also does all these things but has several other important abilities plants don't have. These are locomotion (the ability to get up and walk around), sentience (the use of the five senses to see the world, and the ability to process these through thoughts), and appetites (likes and dislikes, pleasures and pain).

The Thomist viewpoint describes human beings as "rational animals." They do all the things animals do but also have intellect and volition. By intellect, the philosopher means more than just thinking. It's the ability to put thoughts, even *abstract* thoughts, into organized arguments for reasoning. Volition is willpower. It is free will in particular—the ability to exercise your will by choosing that which is morally right (even if it is contrary to your appetites).

Those are important distinctions because it certainly can be argued that animals think about things and make choices. But they do not think about abstracts (like law or math equations), or form reasoned arguments. Another way to say this is that (as far as the evidence shows) animals can't conceptualize and universalize the things they encounter with their senses. To take an example from Aristotle, an animal may identify water and that it must have water to live, but it does not know what water is. You will not see a dog discuss water in its three states, or break it down to the molecular formula of H2O we humans are familiar with. It may not understand that the substance sloshing around in the bowl on the floor is the same substance trickling down the mountain in a stream. And because they lack "the deliberative faculty" (meaning they don't have the ability to decide rationally whether a thing is right or wrong to do), animals don't have volition. They are not moral beings: they do not choose to do things because they are morally right and wrong (mainly because they cannot understand the concept of right or wrong). They process information from their senses and proceed based on their desires and needs.

Here's an example of this organization of life in St. Thomas Aquinas' writing on natural moral law:

> "First, there is present in man the inclination toward the good on the level of the nature which he shares with all substances, inasmuch as each substance desires the preservation of its own existence according to its own nature…"
>
> "Second, there is present in man an inclination toward some more special things, on the level of the nature which he shares with other animals…"
>
> "Third, there is present in man an inclination toward the good that is in accord with the nature of reason, and this is

proper to him." [xlviii]

By the word "proper," Aquinas means particular. Aquinas writes about the souls of animals and plants. It's common in philosophy to use the term "soul" to mean the "first principle of life"—that is, the thing that makes inanimate bodies alive. The soul spoken of in this sense is (in my own simplified terms) that mysterious something that is required to move a body from a dead body to a living one, rather than the theological term for "the image of God" which we discussed earlier.

Medieval philosophers distinguished living things from nonliving things and pointed out that mankind and animal-kind (and plant-kind) share this sort of "soul," or first principle of life. Throughout early and medieval church history there was much discussion among Christian thinkers about the rational faculties of animals. Some argued that animals differ from humans because they lack rationality, the ability to conceptualize and reason with logic. It is this part of the soul that elevates mankind ("the rational animal") above the beasts.

The lack of intellect and volition, two parts of what theology calls "the image of God," are what moves Thomist philosophers to accurately conclude that animals are entirely corporeal beings. I think it's very important to add to this philosophical reasoning the theological truth that the image of God is part of the whole person (not just the intellect or will). In a mysterious, comprehensive way humankind shares in God's image and animal-kind lacks God's image.

Interesting. But what does it matter?

A clear and well-reasoned view of our relation to other living things helps us be more certain in how we treat them. Thomas Aquinas' detailed thoughts, grounded in and extending from Scriptural revelation, carry practical implications in how we relate to real animals in the real world. The Thomist view of a hierarchy to life tells us we should not treat animals like we do rocks (non-life), or like we do trees (plant-life).

This differs from the Cartesian viewpoint (related to the ideas of Descartes), for instance, that animals are just fancy machines, entitled to no respect or care as living things.

It is ironic that the prevailing philosophical viewpoint in our modern world, even among religious people, is deeply rooted in the materialistic philosophy of René Descartes. It was Descartes who propounded the idea of radical separation of the body from the soul. The body, he said, is only a machine that the soul inhabits. One's soul, as later philosophers would paraphrase Descartes' idea, was merely "the ghost in the machine." This differs from the more organic Christian (and Thomist) viewpoint that our soul and body are intertwined, making us into "the image of God." The extreme, dichotomous view of Descartes led him to notoriously characterize an animal as a complete automaton, no different from a music box because it is entirely corporeal. The Christian philosopher, on the other hand, can recognize the "soul" in the corporeal.

Thomist, Augustinian, and Aristotelian Hierarchy of Life[xlix]

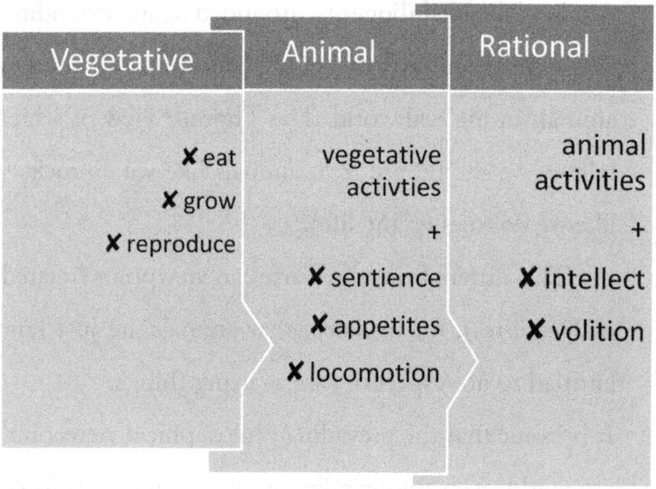

Definitions:

Appetites: likes and dislikes, feeling pleasure or pain.

Intellect: understanding abstract concepts and able to organize them into thoughts, and use those thoughts to reason through logic.

Locomotion: ability to move (walking, running, slithering, etc).

Sentience: sense perceptions (taste, touch, smell, etc) and being aware of the meaning of those perceptions. This also includes imagination: the ability to form images in the mind based on the senses.

Volition: the ability to choose right and wrong, regardless of appetite. Will-power.

There is a special something in all of life, human and animal, which elevates it above non-life (in intrinsic value, abilities, and in how we are morally bound to treat it).

Since his day, so many have moved to complete materialism, denying the existence of the soul at all. There is no ghost at all, many say, only the machine. Thomas Aquinas argued a very different viewpoint, even though he did not believe animals had the same immortal soul as humans do. The Thomist philosopher preserves the Biblical value of living things over non-living things and argues from it a further gradient of thinking and consciousness among living things that matches reality. Lacking a rational soul does not make a creature a mere machine.

Conversely, the Thomist view also tells us we should not treat animals like we do people. The status of animals, in the eyes of early church philosophy, was between man and non-living things in value. It's this view of animal-kind that allows a proper balance in how we relate to them and lines up best with Scriptural teaching.

– IV –
Observations and Conclusions

Animals Are Not Little People

The words of Genesis 1:26 are vital to this study and are worth dwelling on more. *"Then God said, 'Let us make man in our image, after our likeness. And let them have dominion over the fish of the sea and over the birds of the heavens and over the livestock and over all the earth and over every creeping thing that creeps on the earth.'"*

We've seen how God made mankind unique in His own image. This is never said of animalkind. Scriptural teaching, and the historic teaching of the church throughout the ages, shows that people are unique to animals. They are, in God's eyes (and thus in reality), more valuable than animals. From our perspective today, with long years seeped in the humanistic traditions of evolutionary doctrine, this is especially important to remember. *Homo sapiens* are not just another species of animal: God uniquely made us in His image with eternal souls and qualities animals do not share.

> *"Killing an animal is sad. Killing a human is murder."*

In typical blunt, but wordy fashion, Martin Luther addresses this in his commentary on Genesis 1:26. "Moses however here sets before us the striking differences between man and all the animals mentioned; when he affirms that man was created by peculiar counsel and providence of God, whereby he signifies that man is a creature far excelling all other animals, which live incorporeal life; which excellence was more especially prominent while nature was as yet unfallen and uncorrupted. The opinion of Epicurus was that man was created only to eat and to drink. This was not separating man from beasts; for beasts have also their pleasures, and they pursue them with delight. Whereas the sacred text before us forcibly expresses the distinction and separation of man from beast, when it affirms that God took deep thought and certain counsel in forming man; which counsel was taken, not only to form man but

"Christian veterinarians need to lead the way in regaining a well-reasoned and Biblical understanding of the human-animal relationship."

to form him 'in the image and after the likeness of God.' This image of God is a far different thing from the care of the belly and the indulgence of the appetite; for these things beasts well understand and eagerly crave."[1]

Luther, arguing from Scripture, parallels Thomas Aquinas' teaching on animal life with remarkable exactitude. Luther was familiar with Aquinas' writings.

These views sound archaic to modern ears. Today, after the

general acceptance of Darwinism and secularism, atheism has infused with new life the Epicurean ideas Luther spoke against. Atheistic, materialistic, and Epicurean thinking is ubiquitous in our society now. All three philosophies vie against the Christian thinking about the place of mankind and animal-kind in the world. Man today is often seen as little more than a biological machine, whose primary interest is "what to eat and to drink." Humans, a large portion of society claims, are just another type of animal.

In my profession as a veterinarian I hear, again and again, the idea expressed that animals have just as much value as humans. I hear this from "regular" people, not ivory tower philosophers. Some have even told me they think animals are *more* valuable than humans. This is contrary to Christian teaching and thinking because it's based on philosophies contrary to Scripture. So many have grown up in a materialistic milieu since their childhood, and unconsciously espouse flip-flopped thinking about animals. Many cannot express why they think animals are better than people: they just feel that way. They are thinking with their emotions, based on an upside-down view of the world.

Because of the widespread confusion today, Christian veterinarians need to lead the way in regaining a well-reasoned and Biblical understanding of the human-animal relationship. We must be clear (in our thinking

> *"Dogs thrive best when you treat them like their own species, not like furry little human beings."*

and in how we communicate to other people) about our human identity in relation to our animal patients, as much as we are about their value in the eyes of the Creator who loves them. Though animal life is beautiful, and ought to be preserved, human life *is* infinitely more valuable. There is nothing in all creation as important or as beautiful as human life. That's why God could command animal sacrifice in the Old Testament but condemn human sacrifice (Leviticus 18:21). That's why it is OK to euthanize a dog in some settings, but not OK to euthanize a human. Killing an animal is sad. Killing a human is murder. We need to stop thinking of humans as hairless animals.

And the reverse is just as important to remember as we discuss veterinary medicine. We need to stop thinking of animals as hairy humans. There is a widespread tendency toward anthropomorphizing animals, which is bad for both the humans and the animals. We do it in our entertainment, spending half our lives awash in media that presents talking animal protagonists, essentially funny-shaped humans with fur. While this is fun, we have to remember this is not reality. We also do this in everyday conversations, as much in our description of our pets as in the words we use about them, which imply reasons for their behavior that they never could have thought of. Perhaps you've heard the (in my view) wildly inappropriate term "fur babies"? But despite all this fantasy that we project upon animal-kind, animals are not little people.

Treating animals like little people has created genuine health concerns for pets in our confused society. People feed dogs and cats their food, and it gives them pancreatitis and gastroenteritis. People carry their dogs in strollers or on their shoulders all day, giving them muscle atrophy and psychological abnormalities. People let their dogs and cats linger in suffering until they're 19 years old and can't walk and need to be fed through an esophagostomy tube and given dozens of medications because they think of them as they would their grandmother. All of this is *not good for* the animals under our care. Dogs thrive best when you treat them like their own species, not like furry little humans.

This anthropomorphic thinking of animals also has the effect of bringing humanity to the level of animals. If "nature is red in tooth and claw," is it any wonder we see increases in violent behavior in a society flooded with the idea that people are the same as animals? We have men behaving like beasts because we've taught them (whether consciously or subconsciously) that men are *merely* beasts.

This is also where much of the confusion with animal euthanasia comes from—one more visible sign of our modern world's confusion about animal nature. I encounter this regularly in my professional life. I've lost count by now of the many times a client said "if only we could do this in human medicine" or "I wish my grandma could get this done" (or words along those lines) when performing euthanasia on a pet. Phrases like that show the confusion people have about our status as humans, as much as they show the confusion about animal-kind. Euthanasia of an animal is not the same as euthanasia of a person for two important reasons. 1) Animals do not have the image of God. They do not have a soul, and killing them is not the same thing as killing a person. 2) Animals are not morally culpable beings like people are (they lack volition or free will). For a human being, killing another human or killing himself is breaking the 6th Commandment. There are no such moral restrictions for an animal. Confusion about animal-kind in our society leads in actual ways to confusion about mankind as well.

These types of practical problems arise when we approach animal life from a view of materialism. We'd do well to remember the words of that great quipster, G. K. Chesterton. "Darwinianism can be used to back up two mad moralities, but it cannot be used to back up a single sane one. The kinship and competition of all living creatures can be used as a reason for being insanely cruel or insanely sentimental; but not for a healthy love of animals… That you and a tiger are one may be a reason for being tender to a tiger. Or it may be a reason for being cruel as the tiger. It is one way to train the tiger to imitate you, it is a shorter way to imitate the tiger. But in neither case does evolution tell you how to treat a tiger reasonably, that is, to admire his stripes while avoiding his claws. If you want to treat a tiger reasonably, you must go back to the garden of Eden."[li]

The materialistic view that animals and people are just

machines leads to extremes. On the one hand, it leads to the extreme that animal life matters no more than a cell phone: it's fun and useful, but if it breaks who cares. If a dog is just a "ghostless machine" then I can kick it and beat it. On the other hand, this view leads to the extreme that loving an animal more than a child is merely a matter of preference. If I'm the same as Fido, I should care about Fido every bit as much as (or more than) my baby or my grandpa.

"Though animal life is beautiful and ought to be preserved, human life is infinitely more valuable."

It's only the balanced view of Scripture (that animal life is beautiful and holds a special place in creation, but is not above human life) that gives us the right perspective. Only when we accept the teachings of God regarding our animal friends are we free to "admire the tiger's stripes while avoiding his claws."

William Youatt, early pioneer in companion animal and veterinary writer, expressed this balanced outlook well. "The most strenuous advocate, then, for the rights of the brute cannot deny the supremacy of man. They were subjected to our power by him who made us both. The question is, How far does this delegated authority extend?"[lii]

The Bible calls us to wonder at all living things, even to a limited feeling of kinship with them, while at the same time proclaiming the astonishing elevation of man by mere association with

God's image. This is because the wonderful God, who made every living thing, set man to rule them and cares for them with a heart big enough to encompass them all. Christian teaching demands a balanced and humane view of animal-kind in relation to mankind: the gentle and beneficent guard of the shepherd for the beast, beating in the same breast as the compassionate heart of the minister for the man.

As Youatt wrote: "The universal Sovereign, the universal Parent, is bestowing his blessing on his innumerable family. Man, destined for a higher sphere than aught the present world can bestow, receives the first benediction and the most valuable gifts—but not one member of the family is excluded. All are his offspring, all share in his blessing; *the fowl, the cattle, and every beast of the field.*"[liii]

Animal Cruelty

The theological and philosophical teachings about animals should shape a Christian worldview of animal care. We are the shepherds of the animal kingdom. God made us to be their guardians. Good people will show their kind natures by treating animals with gentleness and kindness, just like God does.

One does not have to come to the subject from a religious viewpoint to see that animal cruelty is wrong. "Animals, too, have their own value," writes David Oderberg about the ethics of animal rights. He speaks of the beauty in the animal world that amazes us, as well as the service animals have done for mankind throughout history. "All of this enjoins upon us obligations of care and respect for animals, and a vigilance that we do not repay their service with cruelty and wanton suffering."[liv] Significantly, the context is that animals don't have rights in the same way as people. The argument has philosophical merit but is too big to include in the limited scope of this book.

Lewis' idea that animal nature is shaped by human redemption works in reverse too—the nature of man changes by how he treats animals. If he abuses them, he shapes himself into a cruel and wicked man (just like—surprise, surprise!—Proverbs 12:10 warns). A man who enjoys suffering in any type of life is a wicked person. Abuse of animals is often a prelude to murder because it shows an evil heart that does not care for life and enjoys hurting things. It confirms and solidifies violent behavior. It may not be shocking to learn that studies on the direct correlation between animal abuse and human abuse have been numerous and well-established, starting as early as the 18th century. Domestic violence and animal abuse often go hand in hand in the same families, and people who abuse animals are more likely to commit violent crimes against other humans as well. The social implication is that they bring violence and even tragedy in communities and deterioration to society. We should instead strive to be kind animal owners, who actively promote the health and wellbeing of the animals under our care.

A Darwinian worldview negatively affects the way we view animals in one of two ways—either a "survival of the fittest" mentality that leads to the conclusion we can treat animals however we need to survive, or a sentimental mentality that views animals as our brothers. In bigger words, a naturalistic philosophy leads either to pragmatic brutality or to an illogical form of quasi-animism. And if there is no eternal reward for good deeds, neither of these conclusions gives much motivation to pursue animal wellbeing.

Only a Christian worldview, infused with a sense of redemptive purpose from the Biblical dominion mandate, will allow for a balanced view of concern for animal welfare without the excess of treating animals as people. That's why the early social movements against animal cruelty were populated largely by outspoken Christians (and veterinarians) like William Youatt.

We can see a sort of disinterested, coldly scientific view of animal suffering developed among Enlightenment and proto-Enlightenment medical theorists because of a Darwinian worldview. Thomas Sydenham (1624-1689) was an influential thinker and writer on medicine in his day and a friend of John Locke. He was famous for saying "all diseases could be described as natural history."[lv] His point was that disease is nature's way of "balancing the scales," of eliminating weaker animals so that the strong can survive. The inferred conclusion of this idea is that there's little need for intervention to cure disease (which characterized Sydenham's minimalist medical practice). The extension of this thinking leads to the idea that we probably ought not to meddle with nature's work by preventing disease.

But this is not a Biblical-based medical thought process. The Bible's teaching that disease and suffering and death were all introduced by the fall implies that disease is unnatural and bad. It is part of the work of redeemed Christians to follow their Savior who is making all things new, and relieve suffering. The redeemed veterinarian's work is to reverse the fall by waging war specifically on suffering and disease in animals. And that's why, when we open the history books, we find Christians at the forefront of research and development of the profession of veterinary medicine at its very beginning.

Ending Thoughts

Christians have wonderful reasons to be interested in veterinary medicine and to consider it a noble profession. We believe it a calling by God. He ingrained into us from our creation to be shepherds over the animals around us, to have a kind dominion as gentle rulers. We believe in a tender God who cares for every beast upon this earth, who knows every sparrow that falls to the ground in suffering, and who is grieved by that suffering. We believe in a calling as Christians to follow our magnificent Savior in His glorious task of reversing the effects of sin in this world. This includes fighting the suffering and death we see in the animal world. We have the words of God commanding us to be righteous people instead of cruel ones, characterized by how we take care of the animals in our lives.

I am proud to work in a profession built, to a remarkable

degree, upon the devoted foundational efforts of fellow Christians. They proved with their lives' work that care for animal wellbeing is an honorable pursuit of the man or woman who follows Jesus.

Christianity presents good theological and philosophical reasons to be concerned with the wellbeing of animals. Yet despite this, there are unique challenges that a veterinary practitioner who also professes faith in Christ must face in today's world. The challenges become more accentuated the more serious a Christian veterinarian is about thinking through their faith and taking seriously the Bible's viewpoint on every aspect of their lives. Many of these challenges stem from deeply rooted, not always well thought through, antithetical philosophies of animal life in relation to human life.

The tendency to equate animal life to human life is a particular problem plaguing the profession today. The Christian veterinarian has to be especially careful how to communicate with clients (animal owners) about issues like euthanasia or controversial procedures like abortions or fetotomy. Some procedures which carry moral consequences in human medicine need not be a factor in animal medicine.

I'd counsel any Christian going into the profession to know that they will face moral dilemmas on opposite extremes as they perform their professional duties. A veterinarian today will see, on the one extreme, the irrational client coming to the clinic in a complete emotional breakdown because they consider their pet to be a child. They will see, on the opposite extreme, the cruel client coming to the clinic to have their pet euthanized for convenience's sake because they don't think of him as anything more than a pastime that has now become problematic.

If you elect to pursue a career in animal health, you'll have to know your stance for both situations and all the nuances in between. And the extra challenge for a Christian veterinarian is to shape that response based on sound theological and philosophical convictions from Scripture.

A philosophically rooted Christian veterinarian may be uniquely well-placed to help both clients (the humans) and patients (the animals), in ways non-Christian veterinarians would struggle with. We have greater motivation to care for the clients who come with our patients. We should serve them like Jesus served others—ready to counsel them in grief, ready to assist them in their righteous duty of caring for their pets. We are well suited to offer educated advice on the practical considerations of balancing the cost of care with a patient's well-being (because we know there *can* morally be a balance between these factors). We may more easily advise clients against some strictly cosmetic and unnecessarily cruel practices, like ear cropping or declawing. We have a firm basis for rejecting convenience euthanasia, while at the same time we can recover from sadly needful euthanasia of a patient, knowing we relieved suffering and are morally in the right.

We've only briefly touched on the host of practical difficulties which work outward from the problematic equating of human and animal life, which extends far beyond the veterinary profession. Considering ourselves to be no higher than animals is to forget our moral imperative as human beings to uphold the image of the God who made us unique. And it makes us ready to imitate the animal world in sensual or violent behavior, which for them is natural, but for us is wrong. It also comes to play in many political questions like animal cruelty laws (which are certainly needful) and environmental rules.

I believe Christian veterinarians are uniquely situated to speak to these matters. We should be careful how we speak about people and animals while performing our professional duties. And we should avoid inflammatory language that encourages extreme behavior regarding animals.

After almost 12 years practicing as a veterinarian (not counting my years in the field as a student and technician before that), even after years of feeling burned out and almost quitting it, I can say I'm still happy to be a veterinarian. I am happy to do my part in the relief of animal suffering and feel honored to have worked with the wonderful patients I have seen. I am happy to help my fellow humans become better people by treating the animals in their care. And I'm happy to be in the unique position to work with a balanced understanding to help my human clients and animal patients as equally as possible.

If you are interested in pursuing a career in veterinary medicine, good for you! Be aware of the challenges you'll face, not just practically, but philosophically as well. But also be aware that you're considering joining a noble profession where a Christian man or woman can serve honorably. If you have a veterinary friend, good for you! Understand that their job is hard, from a philosophical, emotional, and practical standpoint. Do what you can to encourage them. If you are a veterinarian currently and a Christian, good for you too! Keep up your hard work with renewed purpose, "you are serving the Lord Christ" (Colossians 3:24b).

Think deeply about your profession in the light of God's Word, and then go out and do it with joy as a service to Jesus, and to the living world He's made. Do your professional work like J.S. Bach, who signed off each of his musical compositions with *soli Deo Gloria*: to the glory of God alone!

About the Author

J. Aaron Gruben grew up in the Southwest and currently lives in Texas with his wife and six children, where he works full time as an emergency veterinarian. A veritable Renaissance man, he is the author of works in multiple genres. His books often highlight historical topics that have become either distorted by political or social bias or have been forgotten by today's general public. When he is not writing or repairing sick animals, Aaron enjoys reading, hiking, acting goofy with his toddlers, and playing a variety of musical instruments.

He also travels to conventions with his publishing company, Post Tenebras Lux Books, which strives to improve lives and revitalize old truths through quality Christian stories and studies. Christ brought Aaron into his camp at 9, and his relationship with his beloved Savior has been the center of his life ever since.

Follow him on Facebook (*facebook.com/authoraarongruben*) and his blog (*nmgrubens.com/blog*) to keep up with new projects and random thoughts.

More Veterinary Resources from J. Aaron Gruben

(Found on posttenebrasluxbooks.com or Amazon)

Fuzzy Logic book series (how to think like a vet)

Animal Anatomy Coloring and Activity Books (Canine & Feline)

Endnotes

Image Credits

Johann Gottlieb Wolstein. Stipple engraving by C. Kohl after G. Kneip. CC BY 4.0 www.creativecommons.org/licenses/by/4.0/. Wellcome Library, London. Wellcome Images images@wellcome.ac.uk www.wellcomeimages.org

Works Cited

[i] Johnson, Alex. "Veterinarians far more likely to die by suicide than other Americans, research shows." Web. December 20, 2018. NBC News. www.nbcnews.com/health/health-news/veterinarians-far-more-likely-die-suicide-other-americans-research-confirms-n950671

[ii] Dunlop, Robert and David Williams. *Veterinary Medicine, an Illustrated History*. Mosby-Year Book, Inc. St. Louis, MI. 1996. P 156

[iii] Heirokles, *Corpus Hippiatricorum Graecorum*. Cited by: McCabe AE. *Hierokles, Hippiatrika, and Byzantine horse-medicine* [B.A. Thesis]. Cambridge, MA: Harvard University; 1993:3 Located at: Library of Colorado State University, Fort Collins, Colorado

[iv] McCabe AE. *Hierokles, Hippiatrika, and Byzantine horse-medicine* [B.A. Thesis]. Cambridge, MA: Harvard University; 1993. Located at: Library of Colorado State University, Fort Collins, Colorado. P 15

[v] Adams JN. *Pelegonius and Latin Veterinary Terminology In the Roman Empire*. Leiden, Netherlands: E.J. Brill; 1995. P 102

[vi] Dunlop 180

[vii] Dunlop 233

[viii] Geerk, Frank. *Paracelsus—Arzt unserer Zeit*. 1992. Wikiquote. Accessed 12/9/19. www.wikiquote.org/wiki/Paracelsus

[ix] Dunlop 234

[x] Dunlop 234

[xi] Dunlop 281

[xii] Larkin, Melinda. "Pioneering a Profession: the Birth of Veterinary Education in the Age of Enlightenment." JAVMA. Accessed 11/7/19. www.avma.org/News/JAVMANews/Pages/110101a.aspx#sidebar
[xiii] Larkin, Melinda. "Pioneering a Profession: the Birth of Veterinary Education in the Age of Enlightenment." JAVMA. Accessed 11/7/19. www.avma.org/News/JAVMANews/Pages/110101a.aspx#sidebar
[xiv] Dunlop 321
[xv] Dunlop 279
[xvi] Dunlop P 297
[xvii] Beal-Preston, Rose. "The Christian Contribution to Medicine." *Triple Helix: Spring*, 2000. Pp 9-14. Christian Medical Fellowship.
[xviii] (Textbox quote) Bråkenhielm, Carl Reinhold. *Linnaeus and homo religious.* Universitet. 2009. P 83
[xix] Moorcroft, William and G. Trebeck. *Travels in the Himalayan Provinces of Hindustan and the Panjab in Ladakh and Kashmir in Peshawar, Kabul, Kunduz, and Bokhara.* William Clowes and Sons. 1841. P XX
[xx] Dunlop 343
[xxi] Dunlop 344
[xxii] Moorcroft XXI
[xxiii] Moorcroft 34
[xxiv] Wochenschr, Dtsch. *William Moorcroft (1767-1825). Veterinarian, explorer in Asia—and spy?* 1991
[xxv] Moorcroft 129
[xxvi] Mushet, David. *The Wrongs of the Animal World.* London: Hatchard, 1839. P xii. Access from Wikipedia, 3/6/21
[xxvii] Youatt, William. *The Obligation and Extent of Humanity to Brutes, Principally Considered with Reference to the Domesticated Animals.* Longman, Orme, Brown, Green, and Longman. London: UK. 1839. P 3
[xxviii] Christian Veterinary Mission. Web. Accessed 4/14/2021. www.cvm.org
[xxix] Youatt 13
[xxx] Lewis, C. S. *The Problem of Pain.* Samizdat University Press. Quebec, Canada. February 2016. P 83
[xxxi] Youatt 8
[xxxii] Smith, Chuck. Proverbs 12:10 commentary on Blue Letter Bible. Accessed 4/14/20201. www.blueletterbible.org/Comm/smith_chuck/c2000_Pro/Pro_011.cfm?a=640010
[xxxiii] Morris, Henry. "Dominion Mandate." N.d. *Institute for Creation Research.* Accessed 11/13/2011. www.icr.org/article/dominion-mandate

[xxxiv] Gruben, J. Aaron and Joy Gruben. *King: A Christian's Call to Imitate Christ's Kingship.* Post Tenebras Lux Books. 2018. P 77
[xxxv] Lewis 89
[xxxvi] Lewis 88
[xxxvii] Piper, John. *Providence.* Crossway: Wheaton, Ill. 2020. P 63
[xxxviii] Calvin, John. Rev. John King translator. *Commentaries on the First Book of Moses Called Genesis, Vol. 1.* Christ Classics Ethereal Library: Grand Rapids, MI. P 53
[xxxix] Gill, John. Anthony Uyl editor. *A Body of Doctrinal Divinity.* "Of the Immortality of the Soul." Devoted Publishing, Woodstock, Ontario. 2016. P 539
[xl] Salisbury, Joyce E. *Do Animals Go to Heaven? Medieval Philosophers Contemplate Heavenly Human Exceptionalism.* Athens Journal of Humanities & Arts. Volume 1, issue 1. January 2014. P 82
[xli] Salisbury 84
[xlii] Romans 8:22-23. ESV
[xliii] Lewis 85-86
[xliv] Lewis 88-89
[xlv] Lewis 89.
[xlvi] Lewis 90
[xlvii] Lewis 91
[xlviii] Aquinas, Thomas. Vernon J. Bourke ed. *The Pocket Aquinas.* Washington Square Press, Inc: New York, NY. 1960. P 198
[xlix] Based on information by Feser, Edward. *David Bentley Hard Jumps the Shark: Why Animals Don't Go to Heaven.* www.thebpublicdiscourse.com April 8, 2015
[l] Luther, Martin. John Nicholas Lenker Ed. *The Precious and Sacred Writings of Martin Luther, Chapter 1: Luther on Genesis.* Christian Classics Ethereal library. Pp 107-108
[li] Chesterton, G.K. *Orthodoxy.* John Lane, London. 1927. Pp 204-205
[lii] Youatt 6
[liii] Youatt 12
[liv] Oderberg, David S. *Applied Ethics: A Non-Consequentialist Approach.* Wily-Blackwell: Hoboken, NJ. 2000. P 140
[lv] Dunlop 319

Made in the USA
Monee, IL
04 November 2026

67380403R00066